™©RiseBright&FIT

1st Edition
© Copyright 2019
All rights reserved
Suzie Lapierre

Self-published in Mississauga, Ontario
Canada
by
Suzie Lapierre

July 29th, 2020

INDEX

Bring
the
Light into
your
Workout

A journey of Self-Commitment

BODY – MIND – SOUL

Suzie Lapierre

I dedicate this book to everyone who is looking to start a journey of commitment into transforming their body, health & spirit.

** **

"Have Faith And Believe In YOUR-SELF,
Anything Can Be Manifested
In Your Life
Thru Consciousness
And Imagination."

DISCLAIMERS

RiseBright&FIT strongly recommends that you consult with your physician before beginning any exercise program. You should be in good physical condition and be able to participate in the exercise. RiseBright&FIT is not a licensed medical care provider and represents that it has no expertise in diagnosing, examining, or treating medical conditions of any kind, or in determining the effect of any specific exercise on a medical condition.

You should understand that when participating in any exercise or exercise program, there is the possibility of physical injury. If you engage in these exercises or exercise programs, you agree that you do so at your own risk, are voluntarily participating in these activities, assume all risk of injury to yourself, and agree to release and discharge RiseBright&FIT from any and all claims or causes of action, known or unknown, arising out of RiseBright&FIT.

The information provided in this book is not intended to be a substitute for professional medical advice, diagnosis or treatment. Never disregard professional medical advice, or delay in seeking it, because of something you have read in this book. Never rely on information in this book in place of seeking professional medical advice.

After reading the content from this book, you are encouraged to review the information carefully with your professional healthcare provider.

PERSONAL DISCLAIMERS
I am not a doctor. The information I provide is based on my personal experience and studies and my experience as a Personal Trainer and Fitness Instructor.

I am not a medical health practitioner or mental health provider and I am not holding myself out to be in any capacity. Rather, I serve as a coach, mentor and guide who help you reach your own health and wellness goals. I aim to accurately represent the information provided in this book and programs. You are acknowledging that you are participating voluntarily in using my information and programs, and you alone are solely and personally responsible for your results. You acknowledge that you take full responsibility for your health, life and well-being in the event that you use the information and programs in this book, I assume no responsibility.

Every effort is made to ensure the accuracy of published information in or through this book and programs; however, the information may inadvertently contain inaccuracies or typographical errors. Every effort has been made to present you with the most accurate, up-to-date information, but because the nature of research constantly evolving, I cannot be held responsible for the accuracy of my content.

RESULTS DISCLAIMERS

I make every effort to ensure that I accurately represent the information and programs in this book and their potential for results. There is no guarantee that you will experience the same results and you accept the risk that the muscle building results, fitness results, competition results and fat loss results differ by individual. I make no guarantees concerning the level of success you may experience, and you accept the risk that results will differ for each individual.

Each individual's health, fitness, and nutrition success depends on his or her background, dedication, desire, and motivation. As with any health-related program or service, your results may vary, and will be based on many variables, including but not limited to, your individual capacity, life experience, unique health and genetic profile, starting point, expertise, and level of commitment.

I cannot guarantee your future results and/or success. Nor can I guarantee that you maintain the results you experience if you do not continue following my programs. I am not responsible for your actions.

The use of my information and programs should be based on your own due diligence and you agree that RiseBright&FIT is not liable for any success or failure of your physique that is directly or indirectly related to the purchase and use of the information and programs of this book.

If this disclaimer scares you or dissuades you from taking action then my information and programs are not for you. However, if this disclaimer inspires you to step up to the plate and make an honest effort at working with the guidance, information and programs I offer in this book, congratulations!

PREFACE

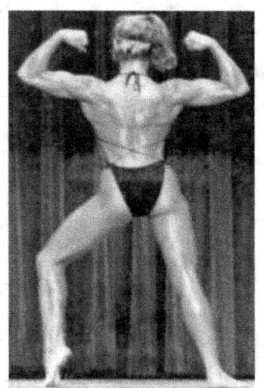 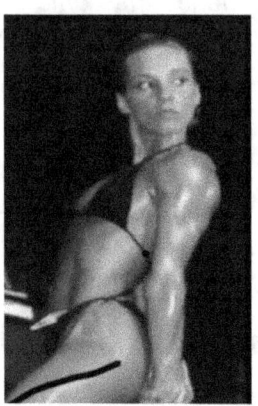

Being in the health and fitness field for over four decades, I've been longing to write this book to share and educate people of all ages who are ready to transform their lives for a better lifestyle, a better YOU, from beginner to advanced.

When I met my coach in my early 20's, I never thought the beginning of this journey would expand to a life-time mission and passion, not only for myself, thus helping others transforming their lives. Thanks to my coach passion, knowledge, patience and persistence for taking the time to educate me on how the body system works, i.e. intensive training and coaching on a daily basis to achieve maximum results. Consequently, his coaching system along with my consistent work and efforts led me to devote myself to bodybuilding competition for five years in Canada and United States. It is with commitments, determination, fortitude, knowledge and love for the sport that I've lived most of my life with these core values, which resulted in a healthy body, mind and soul, now and then.

THE BODY SYSTEM

The following explains how the body system works when engaging yourself in a fitness program of all fitness levels.

We all know that exercise is good for you, but when you understand why, it makes you want to get into the gym a lot easier. Here's an explanation of what happens when you workout, and how it can help you deal with the pains and the gains you'll run into down the line.

The body is a complex machine. We like to think that when we workout we'll immediately feel and look better, it's not always that simple. A lot happens in your body when you first start working out, and the longer you workout the less things change. Here's what you can expect, what's happening, and how you can use that knowledge to improve your workout routine.

What Happens to Your Body When You First Start Exercising

The first thing you notice when you start working out is that you're out of breath and your pulse is high, this is always a bit concerning, but it's perfectly normal. When you first start working out, your body responds by raising your heart rate and causing you to breathe heavy.

While those first few weeks are tough, exercise gets a lot easier as you go along, and it's because your body starts adapting to your workout. Of course, everything in your body is connected, so while you might only feel a difference in your breathing or heart rate at first, it's tied to your muscles as well:

The way you get the oxygen to the muscle fibers is by breathing oxygen into your lungs and then your heart pumps the oxygenated blood into your muscle. So, today you jump on the treadmill for the first time and you run three miles. Your heart rate is high, your breathing is heavy, and you feel crappy. But if you do that every day for three or four weeks, you'll notice that at the same speed your breathing won't be that hard. The reason for this is because your muscle has changed and it's using oxygen a lot better which lowers your heart rate.

Those muscle changes are important, and it's not exactly as simple as you might think. Depending on the type of exercise you're doing your muscles can change in different ways:

For example, in your legs you have two different kinds of muscle: you have fast twitch muscles and slow twitch muscles. The slow twitch muscle has muscle fibers that are better suited for long-duration endurance exercise. The fast twitch muscle has muscle fibers that are better for short, high-intensity bursts. For example, a distance runner would have a lot of slow twitch muscle fibers, on the other hand a sprinter would have more fast twitch muscle fibers.

Let's say we all start at the same baseline where we have half slow twitch muscle fibers and half fast twitch muscle fibers. When you start an exercise program that's about endurance, like jogging, your muscle changes so it has more slow twitch muscles and less fast twitch muscles. This means your muscle can generate force for a longer period of time without fatiguing.

Why tone up?

Life today sees many of us 'sitting' for long periods during the day, every day. Our muscles pay the price: the stiffness of joints and the weakening of muscles that "we sometimes blame on aging" are often a direct effect of inactivity.

Making the effort to have toned muscles will mean you have strong muscles. Strong muscles are firmer, they look better, and they help avoid potentially debilitating bone and joint injuries. Doing strength training exercises can increase your lean body mass (the non-fat parts of your body), which raises your metabolic rate, therefore helping with weight management. Having well-trained muscles also improve your ability to take up and use glucose which reduces your risk of type 2 diabetes.

Why Your Muscles Feel Sore

The awful truth of exercise is that while it can make you feel better over time, you're going to feel bad at the beginning. The reason is that exercise actually damages your muscles:

Someone who has been a couch potato for a while and starts working out will notice that they're sore. What's happening is they're doing very small damage to their muscles each time they work out. It sounds bad, but it's actually good. The muscle responds by repairing itself and that makes the muscle stronger than it was before.

It's not the old motto of "no pain, no gain," though. It's progress and development, and you need to be careful when you're first starting because an injury will likely cause you to break your habit. Thankfully, we know what you should expect to feel when you first start.

So you're sore, and you're weak. That's because the muscle damage causes inflammation and pain. That's a critical part of the muscle adapting and getting stronger. That soreness usually lasts for 24-48 hours and for some people a little bit longer. It's called delayed onset muscle soreness. People should feel it, but it shouldn't make them never go back.

So, watch out for "severe pain".

Minor to moderate pain or soreness is considered normal. Severe pain, however, is considered abnormal, and may be caused by overexertion or poor breathing techniques.

You will experience a little pain, but it's an inevitable step. If it gets to a point where you can't do the exercise again, you need to back off and lower the intensity a bit until your muscles catch up. Take days off in-between exercises or work different groups of muscles. If you do push yourself too hard, take some time to recover and treat yourself right.

Why Exercise Makes You Feel Better

We always hear that exercise makes you feel better in all sorts of ways. From the brain to the lungs, you benefit from a bit of exercise every day. That doesn't really mean anything to you until you actually start exercising though. In addition to everything above, a few other changes you will feel right away that make life a bit easier.

The other thing that happens is your heart gets bigger and stronger. Those are the things that people notice. You're getting these changes in the muscle that actually make exercise feel easier. In addition to your heart rate slowing down and your heart getting bigger and stronger, your blood vessels become more elastic. That's really good. That means your blood pressure can be lower.

Additionally, you're also burning calories and fat, which contributes to weight loss. Your body typically burns calories from carbohydrates for energy first, and then moves onto burning fat as a source of energy. When you burn more calories than you take in, you'll tap into fat for energy and lose weight. If you don't use calories for energy, your body starts to store them as fat cells for an energy reserve.

On top of easier breathing, a lower pulse, lower blood pressure, and everything else, your brain function also improves. Here's why.

Exercise improves oxygen flow to the brain. It also helps the body release hormones that assist in brain cell growth. Additionally, it helps the brain with both learning and memory capabilities. You will feel these improvements quickly, even if you don't see a change in your body.

You can expect to feel healthier and stronger after two to three weeks of exercise (along with a proper nutrition plan). However, you may not see any significant changes in muscle growth or weight loss (depending upon your goals) until after the first few months.

Organically, when you start exercising, you feel better because your brain and body can do more. You're not winded walking up stairs. Your heart rate and blood pressure go down, which decreases your risk for a number of diseases and gives you more energy. Your brain benefits from the added oxygen to help you perform basic tasks easier.

Pick the Right Workout

Depending on your goals, certain workouts are better than others. Since your muscles and body react differently to different workouts, it's important to come up with your goal first, and then choose the workout.

If You Want to Just Maintain a Healthy Lifestyle

If all you want to maintain a healthy lifestyle, your best bet is to work out all your muscles in a few different ways. For most people, the usual recommendation of 30 minutes of moderate intensity workouts a day, including walking, jogging, swimming, or biking, is a good starting point for most people.

Low impact exercises are excellent for keeping yourself in shape without working yourself too hard.

If you don't have a lot of time, exercises like a 5-8 minute full workout or a 20 minute workout make it a bit easier to fit a workout into your schedule. You won't see big fitness gains, but your overall health will remain consistent. Once your body adapts to what you're doing, it doesn't continue to build on that muscle.

One of the things I've learned is that health benefits can come from a lot less than what you need to see the strength and endurance benefits. Someone who goes from nothing to doing about 30 minutes of exercise a day will see a big improvement in

their health and maintain it. Obviously, it gets better if they add more time to that. The benefits kind of plateau. It benefits like better control of blood sugar, lower blood pressure, and lower blood cholesterol, _so those are good things to have plateau._
Once you get going, a few suggestions for balancing your diet with your new workout routine so you can maintain your health.

The best way to support a healthy exercise regimen is to moderately increase carbohydrate intake, in addition to eating foods high in protein and healthy fats. Foods high in _good_ carbs that support a workout program are whole grains, fruits and vegetables. Foods high in healthy fats include avocados, fish, peanut butter, and olive oil, etc. Foods high in protein include chicken, fish, lean beef, dairy products, beans, etc. (Refer to my first book "You will see it when you believe it" for more information on eating healthy sold on amazon.com).

Basically, if you can consistently keep up the 30 or so minutes a day of exercise then you're on the right track to maintaining a healthy lifestyle. You're not going to see big endurance or muscle gains, _but you'll hit the targets needed to improve your health_.

If You Want to Lose Weight

This is a question I've been asked so many times "Suzie, I want to lose weight but I don't know how and where to start?"

Losing weight requires a different approach because you want to work the _slow twitch_ fibers in your muscle more than the _fast twitch_.

When you exercise for a longer duration, you're going to use the slow twitch fibers that are really good at burning fat. If you went and did a couple hundred meter sprints for your workout, it only works the fast muscle fibers, and they use primarily carbohydrates and don't burn that much fat at all.
For example, when you get on an elliptical or treadmill you can push the "fat burning" button, it will be longer and lower intensity because that favors the muscles that are going to burn more fat. So if you do a jog instead of a sprint, you're burning more fat. That

said, it's not all cut and dried. While lower intensity workouts are better at helping you lose weight, you still need to mix it up a little:

It also depends on how many calories you burn. So, you could walk really slowly, but that's burning just fat and you're not burning that many calories. So, there's a balance between whether you burn more fat in the muscle and how many total calories you're burning. Somewhere in the moderate intensity range is probably right. _That said, doing high-intensity interval training will burn more fat because it's so intense that you're burning enough calories to get to the fat._

Therefore, the answer to what workout you should do to burn fat really depends on what you can handle. _A high-intensity interval workout_ will burn the fat after it burns the calories, but it's a lot harder to get into because it's such an intense workout. For many, starting with moderate intensity exercise will ease that process. Moderate intensity has a different meaning for everyone depending on your starting point, but it can range from a brisk walk to swimming. _Moderate exercise means_: your breathing quickens a little, you develop a light sweat after about 10 minutes of exercise, and you can carry on a conversation but can't sing.

Of course, when you're losing weight, you also need to moderate your diet for it to stick because you don't want to take in more calories than you're burning. If you need a little help with motivation, below are tips on how to track your weight loss.
Please refer to my first book "You will see it when you believe it" regarding the 80/20 diet rule and how to apply it. You can find my books on amazon.com.

High Reps or Low Reps for Fat Loss?

This debated topic comes up a lot in the fitness world: Is it better to use light weights and high repetitions or heavy weights and low repetitions for fat loss? The answer is… both!

That answer may seem controversial, but it's accurate. A combination of heavy strength training and high-repetition metabolic conditioning is the most effective and scientifically proven way to lose fat and maintain muscle. Here's why.

Myth: Light weights with high reps will tone muscle and burn fat.

Fact: Light weights with high reps alone don't tone muscle or burn fat.

People often use light weights and high reps exclusively when aiming to lose fat, but this is a huge mistake, especially if you want to have toned muscles, because lifting weights doesn't stimulate muscles enough for fat loss. Focused nutrition and high-intensity interval training (HIIT) take care of fat loss, while strength training will help you keep the muscle you already have. That said, to maintain the most muscle possible, you have to lift weights that are heavy enough to convince your body that it still needs that muscle tissue.

Do: Use light weights and high reps, but not in the traditional sense of weightlifting. Instead, do full-body exercises in a circuit, performing high reps with limited rest. **See my HIIT workouts from pages 87 to 109**.

Myth: Heavy weights build muscle, muscle increase metabolism, so lift heavy to burn fat.

Fact: Heavy weights build strength, which helps you maintain muscle while losing fat.

Lifting heavy weights with low reps won't help you lose much weight, but it will help you maintain hard-earned muscle while losing fat. High reps (12 or more reps per set) build muscular endurance but don't really build strength. Sets in the 3–10 rep range work best for keeping the muscle you already have, then HIIT helps strip away the fat tissue on top of those muscles.

A study from McMaster University scientists found that overweight individuals who lifted weights while dieting lost significantly less muscle mass than subjects who only performed aerobic exercise while following the same diet. The catch: The subjects who lifted weights and the subjects who did cardio lost the same amount of weight overall.

The lesson to learn is that resistance training using moderate to heavy weights gives your body a reason to hold onto muscle tissue. In the end, the weight you lose will be more fat than muscle.

Do: Lift weights 2–3 times per week, using compound exercises like squats, deadlifts, pushups and rows. Do 3–10 reps per set, and stop each set 1–2 reps shy of failure.

Myth: Cardio burns more calories than lifting weights.

Fact: Straight cardio burns more calories during the workout than lifting weights, but HIIT burns more calories overall because it raises your metabolism for several hours after your workout.
The most efficient way to lose fat fast is to create as large a metabolic disturbance as possible during your workouts. In plain English, you want to push your body to its limit with quick bursts of intense exercise followed by periods of incomplete rest. That's the concept behind HIIT, and it's hands-down more effective than traditional cardio for fat loss.

(Look up my HIIT workouts at the end of the book. Pick and choose the workout that suits you best, perform and see results).

THE BIG PAYOFFS

In the end, nutrition has the biggest impact on overall weight loss, but using a combination of strength training (heavy weights, low reps) and HIIT (light weights, high reps) can help you lose more fat and keep more muscle.

To summarize:

Maintain a subtle calorie deficit to ensure you lose weight gradually (and use the MyFitnessPal app to track your calories for better results).

Eat enough protein to maintain muscle (about 1 gram per pound of body weight).

Lift moderate to heavy weights for sets of 3–10 reps 2–3 times per week to maintain muscle mass.

Perform high-intensity interval training 2–3 times per week to stimulate fat loss.

Weight

One way to measure your weight loss progress is to track your weight from week to week. Your weight can fluctuate throughout the day, so it's important to weigh yourself at the same day and time and under the same circumstances. First thing in the morning is usually best.

One drawback to weighing yourself is: your goal is to lose "fat" not "weight." A regular scale won't tell you if you're losing fat or muscle. It also won't tell you if the weight you've gained is fat or muscle.

<u>Let me start off with a few myths</u>:

- Fat weighs more than muscle
- The numbers on the scale tell the full story
- The more calories you cut the more weight you will lose
- You can reduce fat in a specific area (spot reduction)
- Lifting weights will make me look bulky (female)

What is weight loss?

Weight loss is the reduction of overall body weight. This can be voluntary by exercise and nutrition or involuntary by illness.

What is fat loss?

Fat loss is the reduction of fat in the body. This fat is stored in fatty tissues, these are found under the skin, body cavity and in small amounts in our muscles. It is often measured as a percentage versus your overall body weight.

Look for a loss of 1 to 2lbs a week.

Body Fat %

Measuring your body fat percentage is a better indicator of what kind of weight you're losing (muscle or fat).

You can use a Body-Fat Weighing Scale Analyzer to measure your body fat % in the privacy of your home. You'll be able to see an increase or decrease if you measure your body fat consistently.

Some people like to use a skin-fold test with a tool called Calipers to pinch different areas of your body and measure body fat.

As with weighing yourself, measure your body fat at the same day and time and under the same circumstances. Never measure your body fat after exercising.

Look for a loss of .5% body fat a week. (That's POINT 5 percent; not FIVE percent.)

Waist or Abdominal Circumference

Measuring your waist circumference on a weekly basis is another way to track your progress. Use a non-elastic measuring tape and measure either at the narrowest part of the torso (waist circumference) OR at belly button level (abdominal circumference). Choose one and stick to it consistently. And don't pull the measuring tape too tight.

One drawback for this method is that you may not see progress as quickly as you'd like. While you will lose fat around the abdomen, it's more difficult to see progress because this is where the most fat tends to accumulate for the average person.

Clothes/Rings

Lastly, clothes and rings can be a good indicator of weight loss. One drawback is that clothes can stretch. Jeans can be tight after coming out of the dryer but then loosen over time. Rings are a good indicator because they don't change shape or stretch out.

If You Want to Increase Your Strength or Endurance

Strength and endurance training are where things get a bit harder to track. As we noted above, the more you work out, the more your body adapts. That means you need to keep pushing it if you want to see improvements in your strength or endurance. Since muscles grow when you push them too hard, it eventually gets difficult to do that:

Once your muscles start to adapt, what you'll need for anything to happen is "overload." The first time you lift weights that's a lot of overload because you're used to doing nothing. Then over time it gets easier. That's when people increase their weight. They do that to generate the overload to continue the adaptation. That progression is true for lifting weights, or endurance performance, or anything else.

We've talked before about getting over plateaus. It's a combination of overloading your muscles and managing your diet. For weight training, this just means increasing your weights so your muscles continue to adapt. For endurance training, it means upping your mileage or intensity.

When all is said and done, exercise is about finding a good medium. When you know what kind of results you want, and what your reasons are behind exercising, it's a lot easier to actually pick a workout you'll stick to.

Choose Your Reps and Sets

The Most Common Set and Rep Combinations for an Exercise

Below are the most commonly used and prescribed combinations of sets and reps you could do per exercise along with the total amount of volume each one produces.

Also included is the level of <u>intensity</u> each rep range falls into as well as <u>what fitness goal</u> that combination of sets/reps/volume is most ideal for.

- **8 sets x 3 reps = 24 reps**
  High intensity – Heavy weights.
  Most ideal for strength related goals.
- **6 sets x 4 reps = 24 reps**
  High intensity – Heavy weights.
  Most ideal for strength related goals.
- **3 sets x 5 reps = 15 reps**
  High intensity – Heavy weights.
  Most ideal for strength related goals.
- **5 sets x 5 reps = 25 reps**
  High to moderate intensity – Heavy to moderate. weights.
  Most ideal for strength related goals.
- **4 sets x 6 reps = 24 reps**
  High to moderate intensity – Heavy to moderate. weights.
  Equally ideal for increasing strength and building muscle.
- **3 sets x 8 reps = 24 reps**
  Moderate intensity – Moderate weights.
  Most ideal for building muscle and increasing strength.
- **4 sets x 8 reps = 32 reps**
  Moderate intensity – Moderate weights.
  Most ideal for building muscle and increasing strength.
- **3 sets x 10 reps = 30 reps**
  Moderate intensity – Moderate weights.
  Most ideal for building muscle and increasing strength.
- **4 sets x 10 reps = 40 reps**
  Moderate to low intensity – Moderate to low weights. Most ideal for building muscle and increasing strength.

- **2 sets x 12 reps = 24 reps**
  Moderate to low intensity – Moderate to low weights. Most ideal for building muscle and endurance.
- **3 sets x 12 reps = 36 reps**
  Moderate to low intensity – Moderate to low weights. Most ideal for building muscle and improving muscle endurance.
- **2 sets x 15 reps = 30 reps**
  Low intensity – Low weights. Most ideal for muscle endurance.
- **2 sets x 20 reps = 40 reps**
  Low intensity – Low weights. Most ideal for muscle endurance.

As you can see, based on your specific goal and what <u>rep range is most ideal for it</u>, you have quite a few set/rep combinations to choose from for each exercise you do.

As you can also probably tell, there are a few principles these very different combinations have in common. The 2 most worth noting are:

The fewer reps you are doing per set, the more sets you do. And, the more reps you do per set, the fewer sets you do. While this isn't an absolute rule, it is what should be happening the majority of the time.

The total volume being done per exercise is pretty similar despite the different amount of sets/reps being used. For example, 10 of the 13 popular combinations shown above produce between 20-36 reps total. So, most of the time, that's probably how much volume you should end up doing per exercise.

Proper Breathing During Exercise

You may already be familiar with some basic breathing techniques while working out, but our breath can do a lot more than help us lift an extra five pounds. It can affect the overall quality of our workouts, our energy levels, and even our ability to burn fat. So it's important to get it right.

The most common breathing "technique" for working out is, "breathe in on the way down, and breathe out on the pushing phase." For one easy example let's look at bench presses. This technique would have us breathe in before we lower the bar to the chest, and then exhale as the bar is pushed away, then repeat.

Breathing correctly is important while exercising for many reasons. One of which is that it helps with posture. The same muscles that help us with our posture are the ones that also help us respire. Good breath, good posture.

There are two major divisions of breathing: belly breathing and chest breathing. Those who practice yoga and breathing meditation are already familiar with belly breathing. Breaths from the chest are shorter and shallower, which does not allow our lungs to fill properly, which then does not provide our muscles with their needed oxygen. If we can create a larger storage space for oxygen, more will get to our muscles, and we will see we need shorter recovery periods between sets, and an overall increase in energy and stamina. And this all comes back to having good posture and knowing how to breathe properly. Good posture will create the physical space we want by properly positioning our diaphragm in relation to our rib cage. Drawing breath in through the "belly" allows us to take in more breath and fill the diaphragm.

Another division in breathing is breathing in through the nose or in through the mouth. Often, people breathe faster than they should while exercising, or they even hold their breath. And generally, those who are "mouth breathers" have a slightly harder time breathing deeply. Drawing air in through the nasal slows our breath and yet allows us to draw in more oxygen than through the mouth. Studies have also shown that people who are better nasal breathers also have better posture. Again, this can be likened to those who regularly practice yoga, meditation and practice controlling their breath.

There is a technique to practice for breathing. It is a three-to-two ratio. Inhale for a count of three and exhale for a count of two and be able to do this easily while exercising. This can be tried while walking up a flight of stairs or on a treadmill. It's hard at first, but it will help provide the body with the maximum amount of oxygen available to us.

Of course, breathing while lifting heavy weights may not fall into this three-to-two ratio, but by coming back to posture, we can know we are getting greater amounts of oxygen.

Now what about breathing and weight loss? The simple answer is that breathing simply allows us to do more. If we breathe right, we can experience a greater range of motion while exercising, do more exercises in a limited amount of time, and work our bodies harder in a routine because it's being fueled by oxygen.

Breathing can also help us lose weight because proper breathing combats stress, and if our bodies are feeling stressed they go into survival mode, slowing metabolism, storing fat because our body is releasing more cortisol, and preventing us from improving our cardiovascular capacities. If we are breathing right, we are relaxed and our bodies function better.

Resting Between Exercises

Another part of training isn't just doing the exercises, it's resting between the exercises. This comes with experience, but the general rule is, the higher the reps, the shorter the rest. So, if you're doing 15 reps, you might rest about 30 to 60 seconds between exercises. If you're lifting very heavy, say 3 to 6 reps, you may need up to two or more minutes.

When lifting to complete fatigue, it takes an average of two to five minutes for your muscles to rest for the next set. When using lighter weight and more repetitions, it takes between 30 seconds *and a minute for your muscles to rest. For beginners, working to fatigue isn't necessary, and starting out too strong can lead to too much post-exercise soreness.*

Resting Between Workouts

I recommend training each muscle group two to three times a week. But, the number of times you lift each week will depend on your training method. In order for muscles to repair and grow, you'll need about 48 hours of rest between workout sessions. If you're training at a high intensity, take a longer rest.

Choosing Your Weight

Choosing how much weight to lift is often based on how many reps and sets you're doing. The general rule is to lift enough weight that you can only complete the desired number of reps. In other words, you want that last rep to be the very last rep you can do with good form.

However, if you're a beginner or if you have medical or health conditions, you may need to avoid complete fatigue and just find a weight that challenges you at a level you can handle.

So, how do you know how much weight you need to challenge your body?

Tips for Choosing Your Weights

The larger the muscles, the heavier the weight: *The muscles of the glutes, thighs, chest, and back can usually handle heavier weight than the smaller muscles of the shoulders, arms, abs, and calves. So, for example, you may want to use about 15 or 20 pounds for squats and 10 to 15 pounds for chest presses.*

You'll usually lift more weight on a machine than with dumbbells: *With machines, you're usually using both arms or both legs for the exercises while, with dumbbells, each limb works independently. So, if you can handle 30 or 40 pounds on a chest* *press machine, you may only be able to handle 15 or 20 pounds per dumbbell, so half the weight.*

If you're a beginner, it's more important to focus on good form *than it is to lift heavy weights.*

Be ready for trial and error: *It may take several workouts to figure out how much weight you need.*

The easiest way to determine how much weight you should use on each lift is to guess.

Here's How to Start

Pick up a moderate weight and do a warm-up set of the exercise of your choice, aiming for about 10 to 16 repetitions.

For set two, increase your weight by 5 or more pounds and perform your goal number of repetitions. If you can do more than your desired number of reps, you can either pick up a heavy weight and continue, or just make a note of that for your next workout.

In general, you should be lifting enough weight that you can only do the desired reps. You should be struggling by the last rep, but still able to finish it with good form.

Keep in mind that every day is different. Some days you'll lift more weight than others. It's just the way the body works, so listen to it and do your best.

For Women - Getting Muscle Tone Without Getting Big

Unfortunately, most women incorrectly believe that the best way to "get muscle tone without getting too big" is to lift light weights for a high number of repetitions. This is not the right approach. Your fears of getting too big are unfounded and without substance. Lifting light weights for a high number of repetitions builds muscle endurance, not strength, and very limited improvement in muscle tone, if any at all, can be achieved through muscular endurance training. <u>You must increase muscle strength to develop muscle tone</u>.

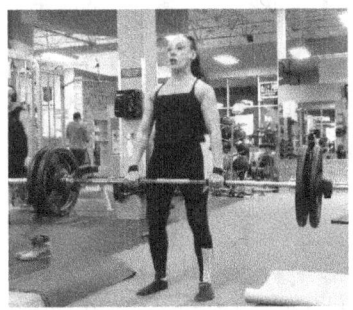
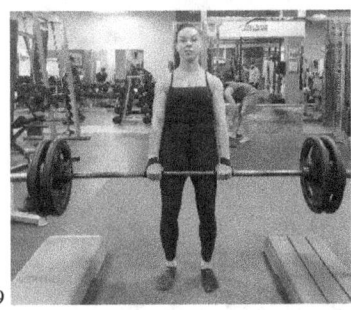

Suzie Lapierre 2019

The solution is to lift heavier weights for fewer repetitions and don't worry about getting too big. It simply won't happen because women are not physiologically disposed toward putting on muscle mass. Blood testosterone levels for women are typically between 15 to 70 nanograms per deciliter. Compare this to men, who have, on average, 300 to 1,000 ng/dL of testosterone in their blood.

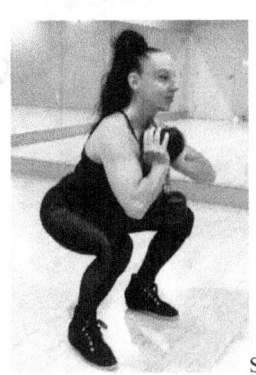
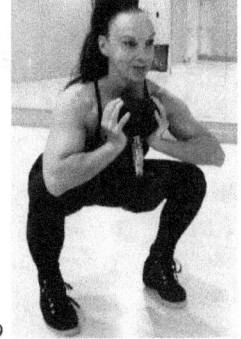

Suzie Lapierre 2019

Testosterone is the key steroid hormone responsible for muscle growth, and women have very little of it. Increasing muscle strength does increase muscle size, there's no doubt about it, but even with a massive testosterone advantage it takes most <u>men</u> enormous amounts of time and dedication to acquire the noticeable levels of muscle mass that so many women are

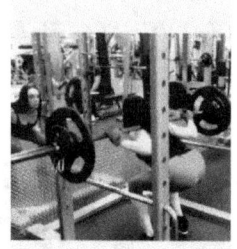

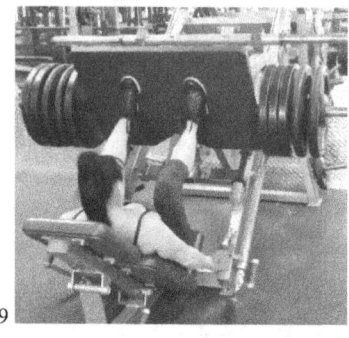

afraid of.
Suzie Lapierre 2019

For a woman, it's true that lifting heavier weights for fewer repetitions will increase your muscle size, but the increase will happen <u>very slowly</u>, and the gains in size will be <u>very small</u>. In fact, the low testosterone levels of women create ideal circumstances for developing the muscle tone that you are looking for.

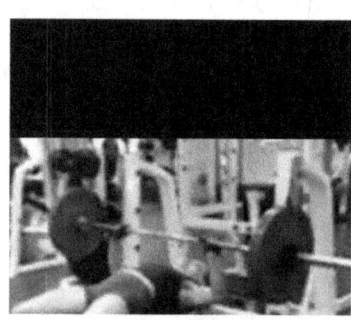

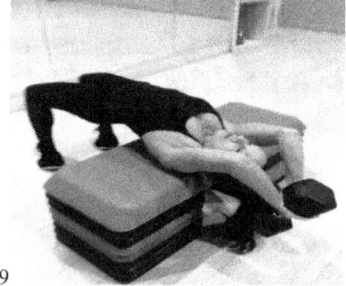

Suzie Lapierre 2019

It allows you to gradually put on small amounts of muscle until you have the toned appearance, without too much size, that you desire, at which point you can modify your strength training program to simply maintain the small amount of muscle mass that you have gained.

There is absolutely no need to fear that you will "get too big," because the size increases happen so slowly that you will be able to halt progress at any size you are happy with, without going too far.

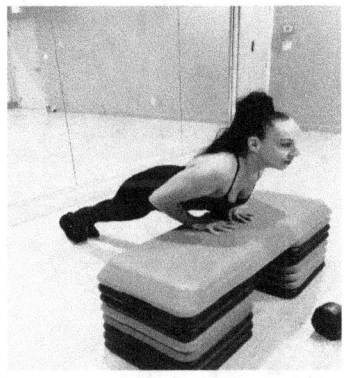
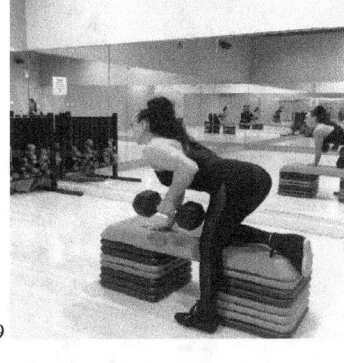

Suzie Lapierre 2019

If you are a woman and you're still not convinced, just try it anyways. Look at yourself in the mirror every day to monitor your muscle tone and size. The worst thing that can happen is that your fears come true, and you are the one woman on the planet that gets huge muscles after a couple of strength building workouts. If we suppose that this does come to pass (it won't), then all you'll need to do is stop lifting weights.

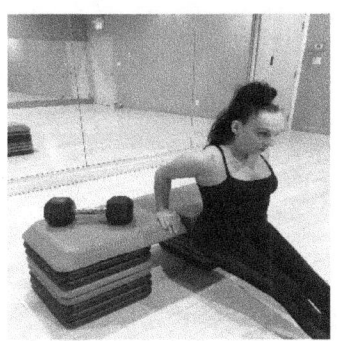
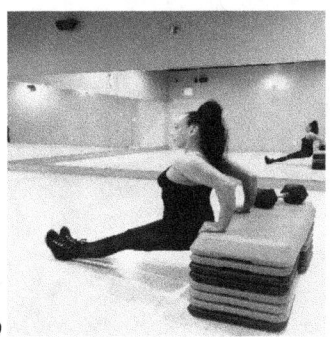

Suzie Lapierre 2019

You will lose all of your size gains in a very short period of time and your muscles will return to their original size (unless, of course, you also happen to be the only person on the planet that does not experience loss of training adaptations after cessation of training). Anyway, you get the point, just try it, you'll be happy with the results.

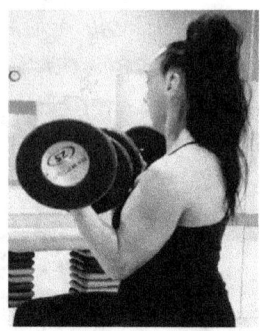 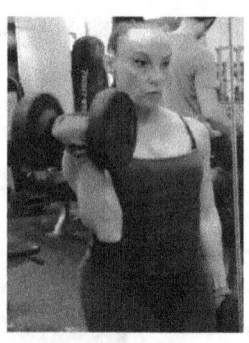

Suzie Lapierre 2019

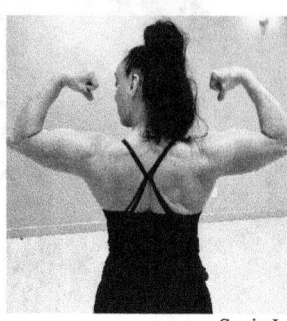 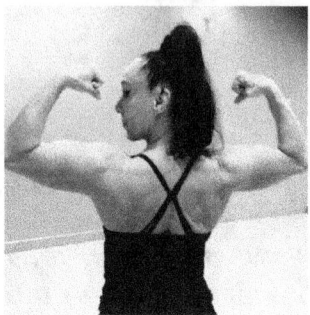

Suzie Lapierre 2019

30

Before & After Pictures

Before and after pictures from a few of my clients.

Selina - 2018 - Before picture

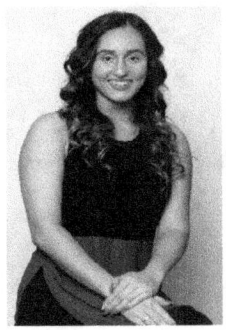

Selina - 2019 - After pictures

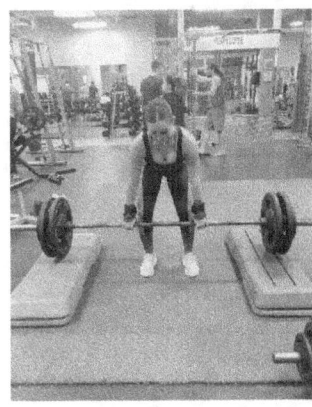
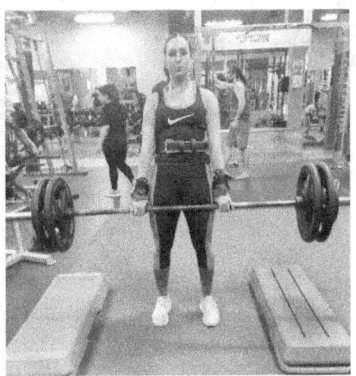

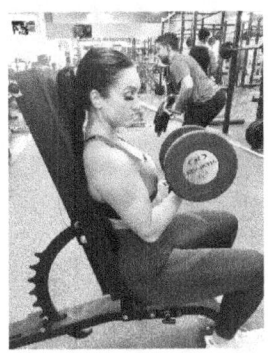
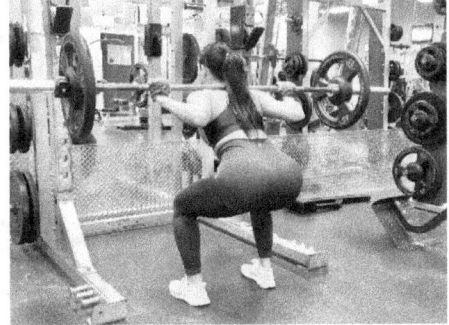

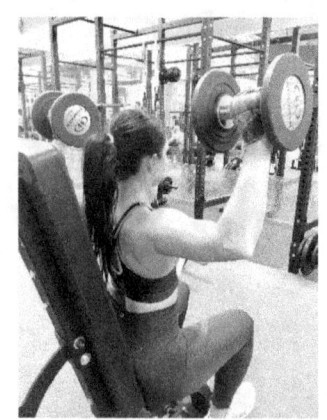
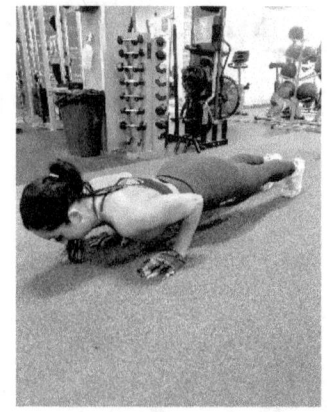
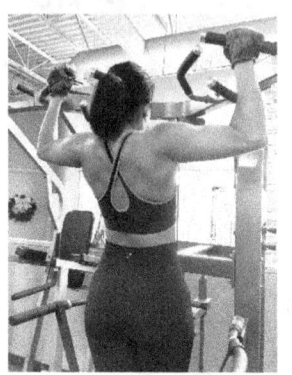
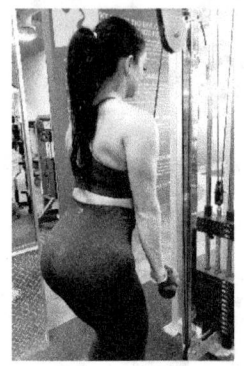

Kathryn – Before pictures – January 2019

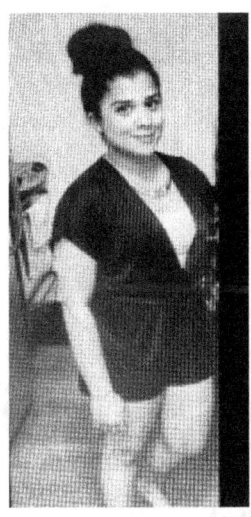

Kathryn – After pictures - February 2020

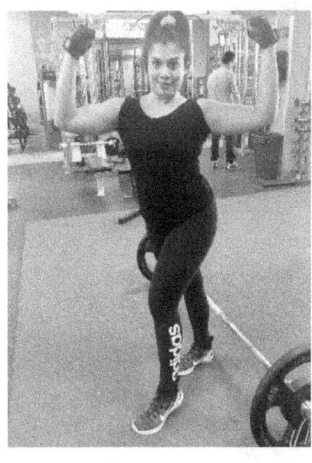

Kathryn – After pictures - February 2020

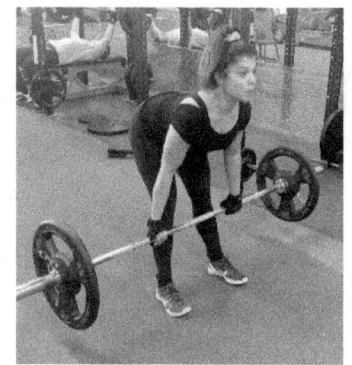
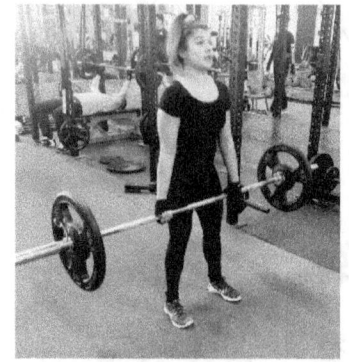

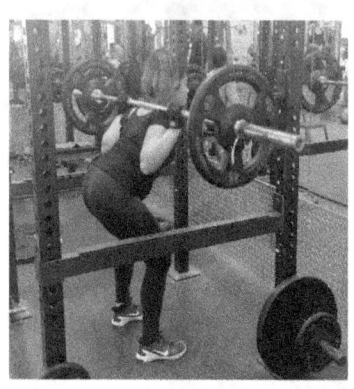
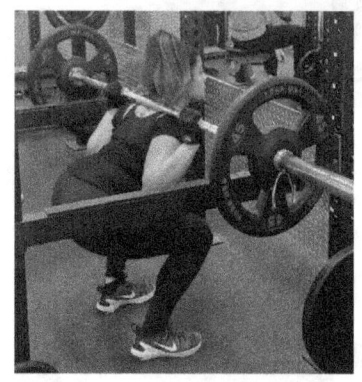

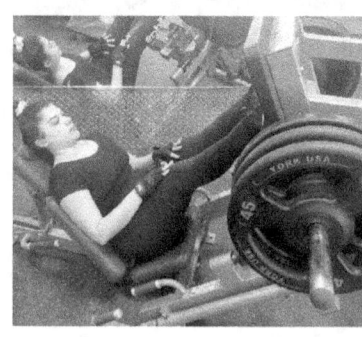
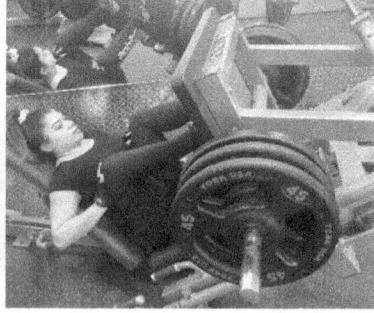

Srini – Before picture - January 2019

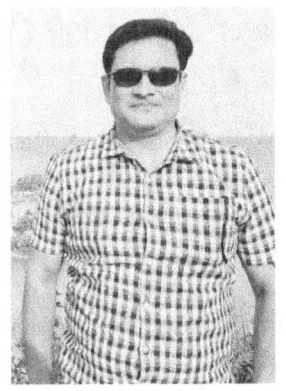

Srini – After pictures - February 2020

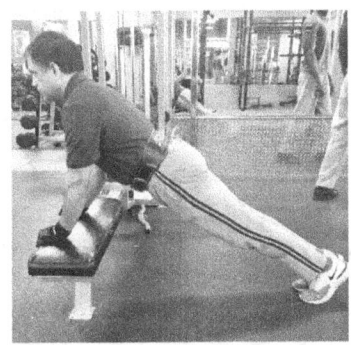 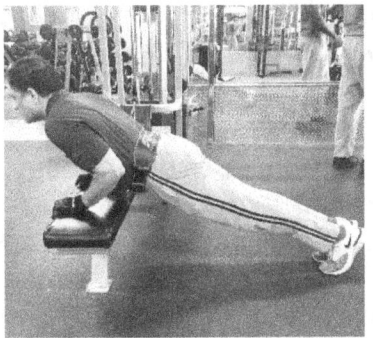

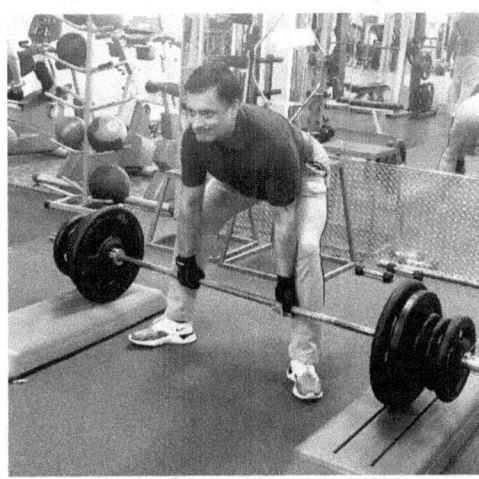 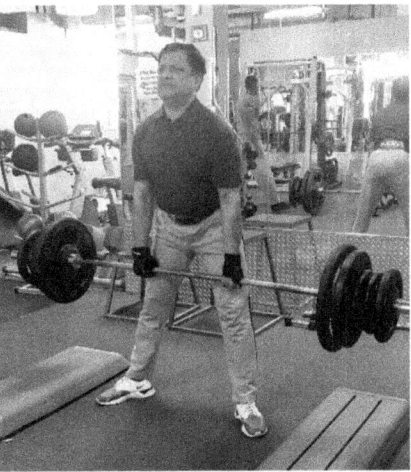

The Benefits of a Group Fitness Class

Group training or group fitness classes have been increasing in popularity over the past decade for good reason.

Whether it's a small group training class based around developing foundational strength or a high intensity bootcamp, gym-goers have many reasons to implement group classes into their weekly routine.

*One of the most important aspects of training is **motivation**. Group fitness classes are a great way to workout alongside friends, coworkers and soon to become friends in a manner that keeps you motivated. Perfect lifting technique or training at the right intensity are not nearly as impactful to your results as being motivated to show up to that day's workout. Group classes make it easy to show up at the gym after a day in the office, with the help of an educated and certified coach to lead your fitness class.*

*In addition to the benefits of being motivated, is **accountability** for your attendance to the program to shape your goals and progress. Training as part of a group class will ensure that your fellow group members and coach will be expecting you at your regularly scheduled timeslot. Missing your one's own workout might feel like it has very little consequence, however, when your group and coach are counting on you those consequences are much greater.*

*Finally, having **fun** with your workouts can be all the difference in seeing the results you want and keeping you coming back for more. Training in a fun atmosphere starts with the instructor. Having a Strength & Conditioning Coach that brings energy and a variety of exercise movements to a class is paramount. Each unique coach will bring something different to the table and have slightly different style of motivating you throughout the session.*

Most gyms offer a growing number of group classes. Whether you want to train with friends or come in on your own but still be motivated by like-minded others, may be the boost your weekly workout routine is looking for.

Here's a few pictures of my regular students who have been committed to my group classes on a weekly basis for many years.

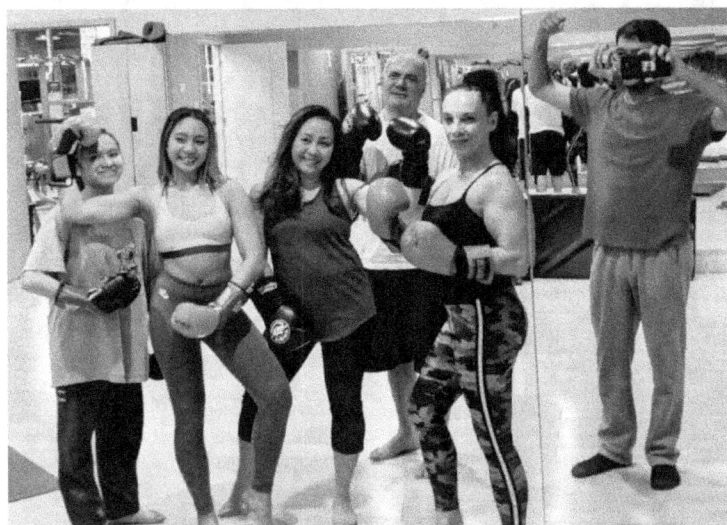

Shaniah, Amanda, Joy, Chris, Me, Anup

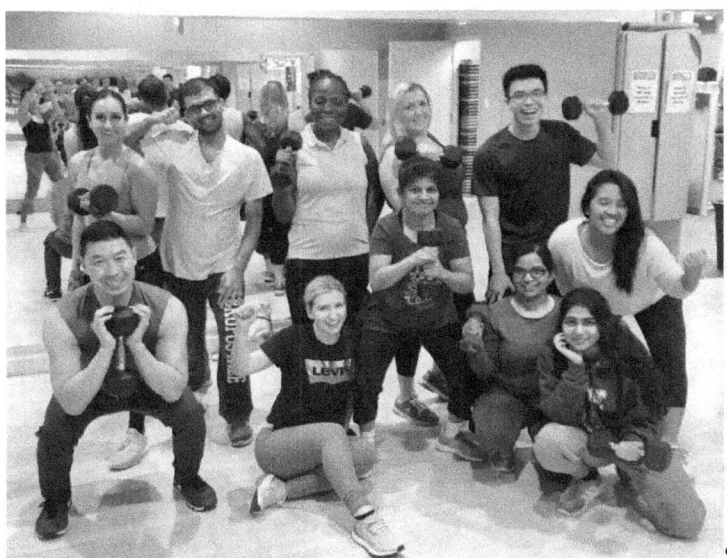

Sylvester, Selina, Anup, Alisia, Dorcas, Shyamala, Cindy, Chris, Sankari, Anysha, Jojo

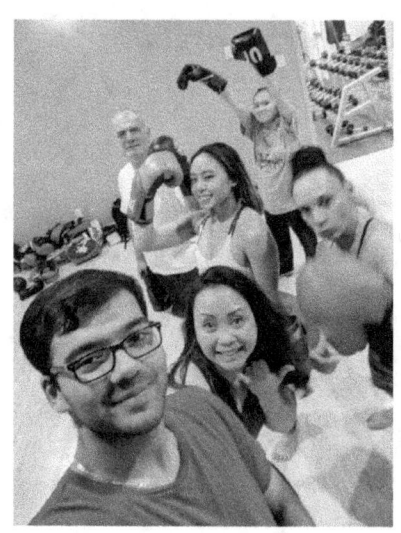

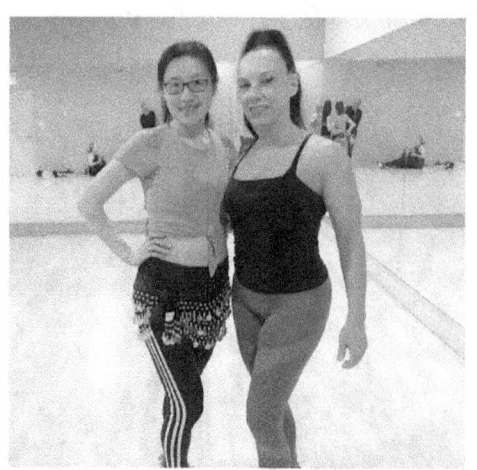

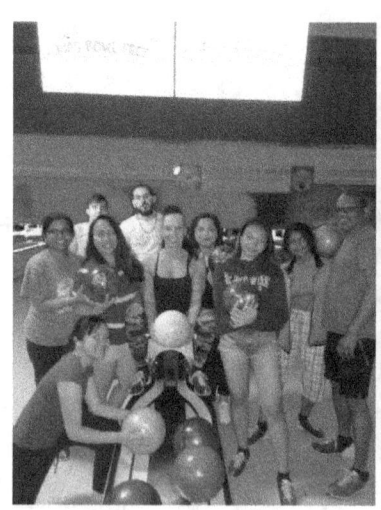

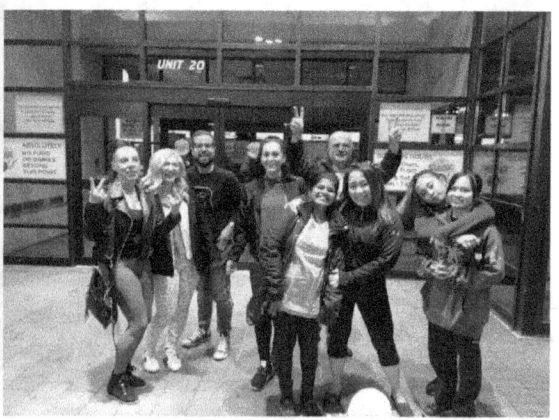

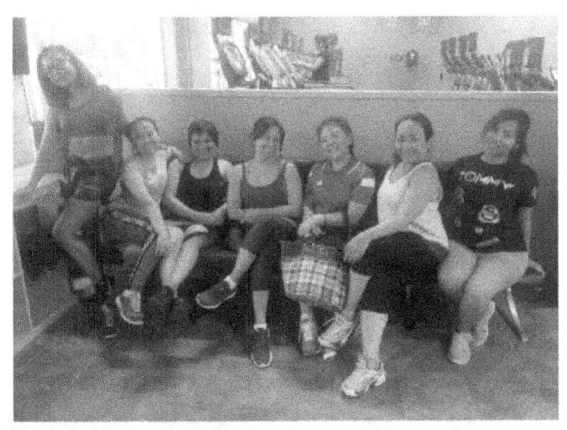

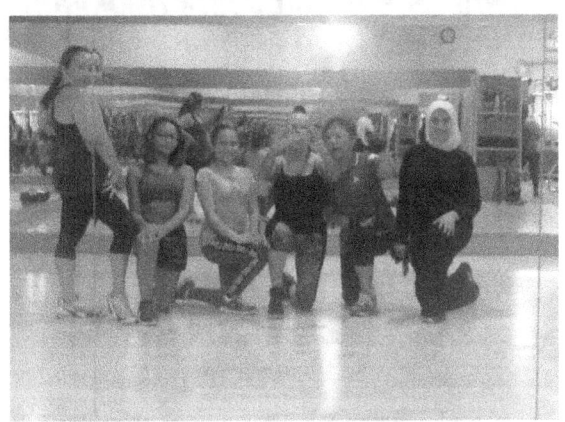

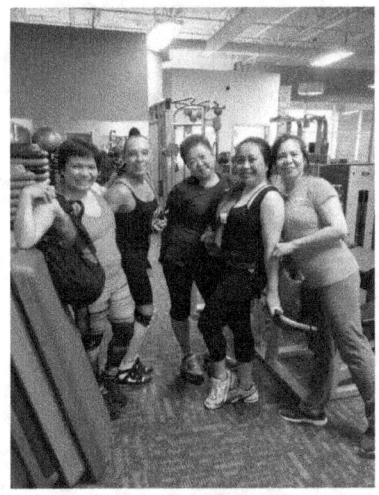

Susie, Me, Louise, Joy, Early

Beginners Strength Training Workout

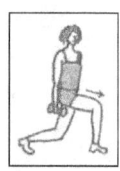

1. *Lunges — to strengthen your hamstrings (back of thigh), quadriceps (front of thigh), gastrocnemius (calf) and gluteus maximus (buttock) muscles.*

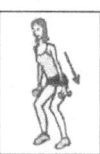

2. *Squats — to strengthen your quadriceps (front of thigh), gluteus maximus (buttock) and soleus (deep calf) muscles.*

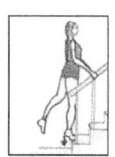

3. *Standing calf raises — to strengthen your gastrocnemius (calf) muscles.*

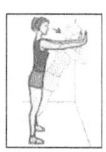

4. *Wall push-ups — to strengthen your chest, arm, shoulder and upper back muscles.*

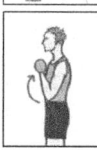

5. *Biceps curl — to strengthen your biceps muscle (at the front of your upper arm).*

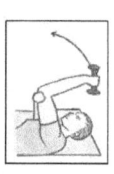

6. *Triceps extension — to strengthen your triceps muscle (at the back of your upper arm).*

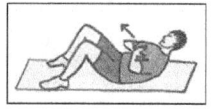

7. *Abdominal crunches — to strengthen your rectus abdominus muscles (at the front of your abdomen).*

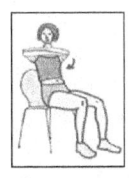

8. Seated abdominal twists — to strengthen your oblique abdominal muscles (at the sides of your abdomen) and your rectus abdominus muscles (at the front of your abdomen).

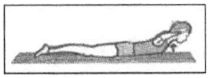

9. Back extensions — to strengthen your upper and middle back muscles.

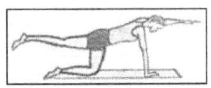

10. Quad knee and arm extension — to strengthen your upper, middle and lower back muscles.

10 Basic Free Weights Exercises For Women

1. Single arm row - *Targets: Back, biceps*

Do: 2 sets of 8-10 reps on left side with a 90-sec rest. Change sides.

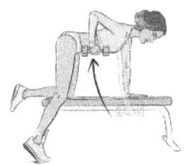

(a) Begin with your right hand and right knee on a bench, your left foot stepped out wide and a dumbbell in your left hand, hanging down.

(b) With your back in a neutral position, and left knee soft, drive left elbow up, lifting the dumbbell to your torso. Lower back to start.

2. Dumbbell chest press - *Targets: Chest, triceps*

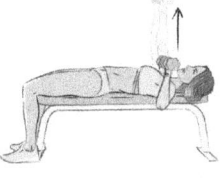

Do: 3 sets of 13-15 reps.

(a) Lie on your back on a bench holding dumbbells with arms straight up over your chest. Bend the elbows slowly, bringing the dumbbells in a straight line down to either side of your chest.

(b) Without pausing, drive your arms back up. Repeat.

3. Split squat - *Targets: Quads, glutes, adductors*

Do: 3 sets of 10-12 reps on each leg. Start with your weaker leg.

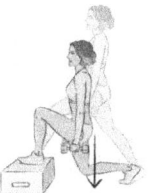

(a) With feet and hips facing forwards, start with one foot raised on a step and your other leg a stride behind you.

(b) Holding dumbbells, slowly lunge forwards, keeping the knee in line with the toe. Without stopping at the bottom, push back up to the start position. Now swap legs.

4. Seated shoulder press - *Targets: Shoulders*

Do: 3 sets of 13-15 reps. If you only make it to 11, use a lighter weight. If you smash 15, use a heavier weight.

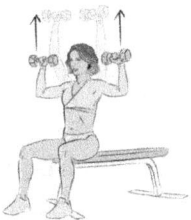

(a) Sitting upright on a bench, start with dumbbells held straight above your head. Slowly bend your elbows and lower dumbbells until they are in line with your shoulders.

(b) Without stopping, drive straight back up to the start position.

5. Hip thrust - *Targets: Glutes*

Do: 3 sets of 15-20 reps. Use a 20kg barbell and 5kg weights on each side.

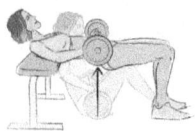

(a) Sit on the floor, back against a bench. Roll the barbell onto the front of your hips. With knees bent, shoulders on the bench, drive hips off the floor until your back is parallel.

(b) Slowly lower your hips downwards, then drive back up again. And repeat.

6. Deadlift - *Targets: Back, hamstrings, glutes*

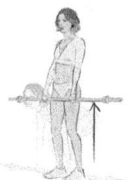

Do: 3 sets of 10-12 reps.

(a) Place an Olympic bar (minus any weights) on the floor and stand with feet hip-width apart. Grip with hands a little wider than your feet. Keep your bottom low, chest up and back flat.

(b) Driving with legs, stand up straight, shoulders back, arms straight down. Keep bar close to your body and return to the floor; <u>maintain a flat back</u>.

7. Step ups - *Targets: Legs, glutes*

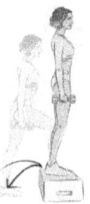

Do: 3 sets of 10-12 reps on each leg.

(a) Start with your weaker leg on a step or box and, with or without dumbbells in your hands, step onto it.

(b) Without pausing at the top, lower back to the start position, leaving your start foot on the box and then stepping straight back up on the same leg. Once you have completed 10-12 reps, switch legs.

8. Seated bicep curls - *Targets: Biceps*

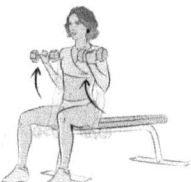

Do: 3 sets of 10 reps.

(a) Sit upright on a bench holding dumbbells, arms down by your sides, palms facing forwards. Bend arms at the elbow, keeping your upper arms tucked in on the side of your rib cage and shoulders still until the dumbbells almost reach them.

(b) Slowly lower (3-4 seconds) the dumbbell back down to the start position. Avoid 'locking' the elbow at the bottom.

9. Lying tricep extension - *Targets: Triceps*

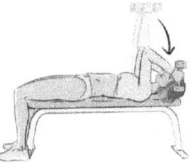

Do: 3 sets of 10 reps.

(a) Lie flat on your back on a bench with dumbbells in hands and arms 90° to your body, above chest. Keeping your shoulders still, slowly bend from the elbows, lowering the dumbbells down until they are next to your ears.

(b) Without pausing at the bottom, straighten your arms back to the start position. Repeat.

10. Seated ball crunch - *Targets: Abs*

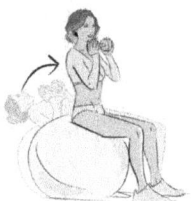

Do: 3 sets of 15-20 reps.

(a) Sitting on a swiss ball, hold a dumbbell against your chest. Slowly lean back until your back is parallel to the floor.

(b) Curl all the way up to a seated position, exhaling and squeezing your abs as you reach the top.

Special Bodybuilding Workout Routines For Men and Women

There are plenty of workout routines out there for men and women, so what is it about these routines that are so special? Well, they are tailor-made to each unique individual, rather than covering a broad demographic.

*Basically, **each routine is designed towards an individual's ability levels and fitness levels in the gym**.*

It wouldn't be much use being very fit and healthy, with many years of training under your belt, following a workout routine that is aimed at complete beginners. You'll already know what you're doing and find the routine far too easy. On the other hand, if you are looking for a new and challenging workout routine, you can follow my advanced program and will enjoy great results.

With that in mind, here are the three routines to try the next time you're in the gym depending on your unique level of fitness:

Beginner Full Body Workout Routine

To start with, let's take a look at a beginner workout routine.

This workout isn't too difficult; though, for those new to health and fitness, it will certainly prove challenging.

Day 1: Chest, Back, Shoulders, Legs, Biceps, Triceps

8. Chest – Dumbbell Bench Press – 4 sets of 8 reps
9. Back – Cable Lat pulldown – 4 sets of 10 reps
10. Shoulders – Seated Dumbbell Press – 4 sets of 10 reps
11. Legs – Leg Extension machine – 4 sets of 10 reps

12. Biceps – Barbell Bicep Curl – 3 sets of 10 reps
13. Triceps – Cable Triceps Rope Pushdown – 3 sets of 15 reps

Day 2: Legs, Triceps, Biceps, Chest, Back, Shoulder

- Legs – Leg Press Machine – 4 sets of 8 reps
- Triceps – Seated Overhead Dumbbell Extension – 3 sets of 20 reps
- Biceps – Barbell Curl – 4 sets of 10 reps
- Chest – Barbell Chest Press – 4 sets of 10 reps
- Back – Bend over T-Bar Row – 4 sets of 10 reps
- Shoulders – Side Lateral Raise – 3 sets of 20 reps

Day 3: Shoulders, Back, Chest, Legs, Triceps, Biceps

- Shoulders – Barbell Upright Row – 3 sets of 15 reps
- Back – Cable Close-Grip Pulldown – 4 sets of 12 reps
- Chest – Cable Fly – 4 sets of 10 reps
- Legs – Lunge – 3 sets of 10 reps per leg
- Triceps – Flat Bench Barbell Skullcrushers – 3 sets of 15 reps
- Biceps – Hammer Curl – 3 sets of 12 reps

Intermediate Workout Split Routine

This next workout is ideal for those of you who are advanced enough to challenge yourselves in the gym without going crazy.

*This workout routine will help you burn a steady amount of fat without burning yourself out in the process. It is a typical **5 day split** that will generate impressive muscle gains.*

Day 1: Chest, Shoulders and Triceps

Chest

- Dumbbell Bench Press – 3 sets of 10, 10, 8 (adding weight) reps
- Incline Dumbbell Bench Press – 3 sets of 10 reps
- Chest Dip – 3 sets of MAX reps

Triceps

- Flat bench Barbell Skullcrushers – 3 sets of 8-10 Reps
- One Arm Dumbbell Extension – 3 sets of 10 reps
- Tricep Extension – 3 sets of 10 reps

Shoulders

- Barbell Front Raise – 4 sets of 12 reps
- Dumbbell Lateral Raise – 4 sets of 15, 12, 8, 8 (adding weight) reps

Day 2: Back and Biceps

Back

- Wide Grip Pull-Up 3 sets of MAX reps
- Cable Lat Pull Down – 3 sets of 10 reps
- Straight Arm Lat Pull Down – 3 sets of 10 reps
- Dumbbell Reverse Fly – 3 sets of 10 reps
- Bent over Row – 3 sets of 8-10 reps

Biceps

- Standing Barbell Curl – 3 sets of 8-10 reps
- Preacher Curl – 3 sets of 10 reps
- Incline Dumbbell Curl – 3 sets of 10 reps

Day 3: Legs

Quads, Glutes and Hamstrings

- Squat – 4 sets of 10,10,8,8 reps
- Dumbbell Lunge – 3 sets of 8 on each leg
- 45 Degree Leg Press – 3 sets of 12 reps
- Leg Curl – 3 sets of 15 reps
- Leg Extension – 3 sets of 15 reps

Calves

- Standing Calf Raise – 5 sets of 10,8,8,8,6 (heavy)reps
- Seated Calf Raise – 5 sets of 15 (light) reps

Day 4: Shoulders, chest, and Triceps

Chest

- Barbell Bench Press – 3 sets of 10, 10, 8 reps
- Dumbbell Fly – 3 sets of 10 reps
- Cable Crossover – 3 sets of 10 reps

Triceps

- Close Grip Bench Press – 4 sets of 10, 10, 8, 6 reps
- Lying Dumbbell Extension – 3 sets of 10 reps
- Tricep Kickback – 3 sets of 10 reps

Shoulders

- Seated Dumbbell Press – 4 sets of 10, 10, 8, 8 reps
- One Arm Cable Lateral Raise – 3 sets of 12 reps

Note: Every second week superset bench press and dumbbell flys. Crossovers: Ultra slow rep timing with 2 second pause and squeeze at the top of the movement.

Day 5: Back and Biceps

Back

- Seated Row – 4 sets of 10 reps
- Bent Over Barbell Row – 3 sets of 10 reps
- Bent Over Dumbbell Row – 3 sets of 12 reps
- Seated Cable Pull Down – 3 sets of 8-10 reps

Biceps

- Cable Curl – 4 sets of 8-10 reps
- Concentration Curl – 3 sets of 10 reps
- Reverse Barbell Curl – 3 sets of 10 reps

Advanced Workout Split Routine

Now it's time for us to take a look at the more advanced workout routine. It is high intensity, includes a lot of heavy lifting, and you should aim for minimal rest between sets.

*Here you will be training for **6 days per week, with just one day of recovery**. It may sound brutal, but if you stick with it you will soon be reaping the rewards of an incredible physique.*

Day 1: Chest & Back

- Barbell Bench Press – work up to a 5 rep max for the day
  - Set 1 at 50% – 1 set of 5 reps
  - Set 2 at 60% – 1 set of 5 reps
  - Set 3 at 70% – 1 set of 5 reps
  - Set 4 at 80% – 1 set of 5 reps
  - Set 5 at 90% – 1 set of 5 reps
  - Set 6 at 100% – 1 set of 5 reps
  - **Set %**: relates to the weight you are lifting in a given exercise, expressed as the percentage of your known 1RM (% of 1RM or 1-Rep Max), e.g., if you are performing bench press with 100kg, and know your 1RM is 110kg, then the load is 90%. You can calculate it online.
- Incline Dumbbell Press – 3 sets of 6-8 reps
- Dip – 3 sets of 6-10 reps
- Pullup – 3 sets of 5-8 reps
- Pendlay Row – 3 sets of 6-10 reps
- Cable Lat Pulldown – 3 sets of 6-10 reps

Day 2: Legs

- Squat: work up to a 5 rep max for the day
  - Set 1 at **50%** – 1 set of 5 reps
  - Set 2 at **60%** – 1 set of 5 reps
  - Set 3 at **70%** – 1 set of 5 reps
  - Set 4 at **80%** – 1 set of 5 reps
  - Set 5 at **90%** – 1 set of 5 reps

- o Set 6 at **100%** – 1 set of 5 reps
- o **Set %:** relates to the weight you are lifting in a given exercise, expressed as the percentage of your known 1RM (% of 1RM or 1-Rep Max), e.g., if you are performing bench press with 100kg, and know your 1RM is 110kg, then the load is 90%. You can calculate it online.
- Leg Press – 3 sets of 6-10 reps
- Stiff-Legged Deadlift – 5 sets of 5 reps
- Hamstring Curl – 3 sets of 6-8 reps
- Calf-Raise – 5 sets of 10 reps

Day 3: Shoulders & Biceps

- Military Press (Front and Back of the Head) – 3 sets of 6-8
- Lateral Raise – 5 sets of 10 reps
- Barbell Curl – 5 sets of 6-10 reps
- Dumbbell Curl – 3 sets of 6-10 reps

Day 4: Rest

It's your rest day. Rest your muscles to prepare for the next round of training.

Day 5: Chest, Shoulders, & Triceps

- Flat Bench Dumbbell Press – 5 sets of 20-6 (Pyramiding) reps
- Incline Dumbbell Press – 3 sets of 6-10 reps
- Chest Press Machine – 3 sets of 10 reps
- Cable Fly – 3 sets of 12-15 reps
- Lateral Raise – 5 sets of 15-20 reps
- Reverse-Grip Pull-Down – 5 sets of 15-20 reps
- Close Grip Bench Press – 3 sets of 10, 10, 8, 6 reps
- Lying Dumbbell Extension – 2 sets of 10 reps
- Tricep Kickback – 2 sets of 10 rep

Day 6: Back & Biceps

- Barbell Row – 5 sets of 20-8 (Pyramiding) reps
- Barbell Shrug – 3 sets of 15-20 reps
- Rack Deadlift – 3 sets of 10-12 reps
- Pullup – 3 sets of 6-10 reps
- Cable Pulldown – 3 sets of 6-10 reps
- Standing Barbell Curl – 2 sets of 8-10 reps

- <u>Preacher Curl</u> – 2 sets of 10 reps
- <u>Incline Dumbbell Curl</u> – 2 sets of 10 reps

<u>Day 7</u>: Legs

- <u>Front Squat</u> – 5 sets of 20-8 (Pyramiding) reps
- <u>Leg Extension</u> – 5 sets of 10 reps
- <u>Hamstring Curl</u> – 5 sets of 6-10 reps
- <u>Seated Calf Raise</u> – 5 sets of 6-10 reps
- <u>Standing Calf Raise</u> – 3 sets of 8-12 reps

Boost Your Exercise Routine With Group Fitness Classes

I would like to add an important point about group fitness classes.

I've been instructing group classes for at least two decades and believe me I always notice a motivation boost when people join my group classes.

Let's be honest, some days you just don't feel like exercising. Whether you run, cycle or walk, sometimes you're just not motivated to get out there. You have all kinds of excuses: It's hot, it's raining, it's cold or I have too much work to do are just some of them. Even professional athletes feel that way. That's because your exercise routine can be downright boring. If getting motivated to exercise is your challenge, perhaps you should consider joining a group to boost your exercise routine. It may be just the kind of motivation you need to get out the door. Group fitness classes keep you accountable, they're fun, you meet new people and they motivate you to reach new goals. A good instructor or group leader can make a big difference, too, in helping you become more fit. In the long run, fitness means a better quality of life. People who exercise live longer, they need fewer medications and they can enjoy physical activities late into their lives.

Benefits of group fitness classes

There are group fitness classes for any interest you may have, from yoga to walking, running, cycling, bootcamp, Zumba, etc. You're sure to find like-minded people because of community's focus on healthy living. Here are some benefits you may find from group fitness classes:

> ➤ *Great for beginners. Most people know exercise is good for them, but they don't know where to start. It can be intimidating starting and exercise class. But group fitness*

classes frequently offer beginner-level courses that help people start safely and effectively.

➤ *You might join a fitness class with friends or at the urging of an instructor. So, when you don't show, they're going to ask you why. On days you don't feel like exercising, sometimes group expectations might be the trick that gets you going. Sometimes, group fitness classes track your progress and that keeps you accountable to a schedule, too.*

➤ *Boredom is a big reason why many people quit an exercise program. Fitness classes often vary the program to keep things interesting, perhaps by rotating instructors or including music with the workouts. Joining other people with the same fitness goals can also keep things interesting as you make new friends.*

➤ *Social connections. You might enjoy signing up for group fitness classes with friends who will keep you motivated. You will likely meet other people who share the same interests, whether it's social or business-related.*

High Intensity Interval Training (HIIT)

What is HIIT?

During HIIT, you give max effort, meaning you work at 100% training capacity, for short, intense bursts of movement, followed by a short period of rest. You repeat this process several times (in "intervals") for a fast and efficient workout that makes you break a sweat and gets your heart racing. It's excellent for people who don't have a ton of time to devote to the gym, as it helps you burn more fat in less time spent.

Why does HIIT work so well? One of the main reasons HIIT works better than other types of aerobic exercise is because it demands more of the body even once you've finished. Research has found that past the point of activity, high-intensity interval training still leaves its imprint. This could help explain the many documented positive side effects of HIIT.

The Benefits of HIIT

Repeatedly, science has found that when it comes to improving your body composition (the amount of fat and muscle you're carrying for your body weight), HIIT might be your greatest ally. In one study with overweight women, researchers compared participants doing HIIT to participants doing moderate intensity continuous training (MICT). While both groups experienced health benefits, the former came out on top regarding body composition, resting heart rate, ventilatory threshold and maximal oxygen uptake. Further research has confirmed that high-intensity training helps improve your aerobic capacity, fat loss and overall body composition for both men and women.

HIIT truly is for everyone, too. One study looked specifically at people who had received a heart transplant and the effect that HIIT had on them, in comparison to continuous moderate training. Overall, HIIT had a bigger positive impact on aerobic capacity, physical fitness and rates of depression.

A Practical Application

Let's not forget that with high-intensity training, you can get a total-body workout in less than 30 minutes. You can do it anywhere, in a hotel, at school, at your office, and with no equipment whatsoever. You can incorporate kettlebells, dumbbells, medicine balls, barbells or other pieces of gym equipment; but it's certainly not a necessity. You can get a perfectly effective HIIT session in with nothing but bodyweight exercises: push-ups, sit-ups, lunges, squats, burpees, jumping jacks and so on.

The only thing that matters is that you're switching between moments of extreme effort and rest. To make it easier on you, set a timer so you know you're devoting adequate time to both.

Staying fit doesn't have to be time-consuming. If you can spare even 20 minutes, you can take better care of your body.

HIIT Workouts for Everyone

The following illustrated exercises are included in my HIIT workouts ahead. You can also view the performed technique videos online.

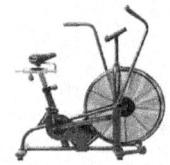 Air Bike

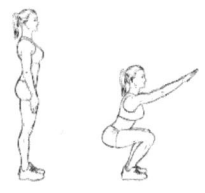 Air Squat

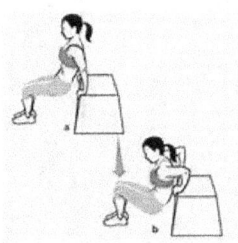 Arms Dip

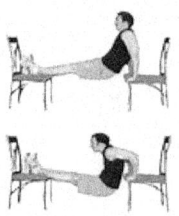

Arms Dip

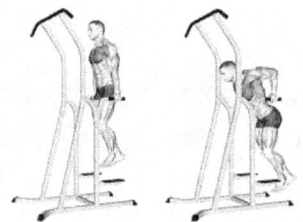

Arms Dip

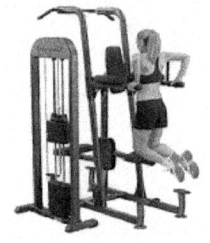

Assisted Arms Dip

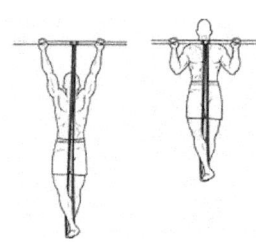

Assissted Pull-Up with Resistance Band

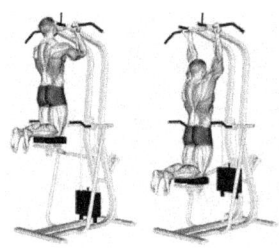

Assisted Pull-Up Machine

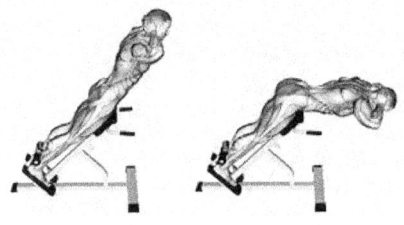

Back Extension

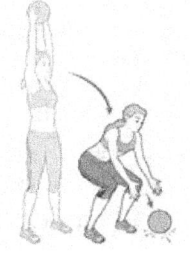

Ball Slam

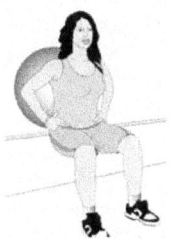

Ball Squat

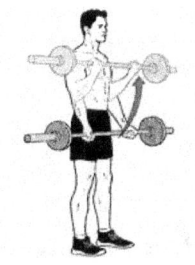

Barbell Arms Curl

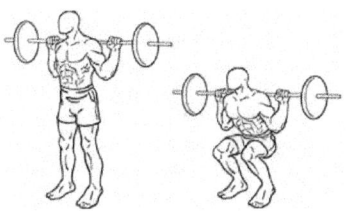

Barbell Back Squat

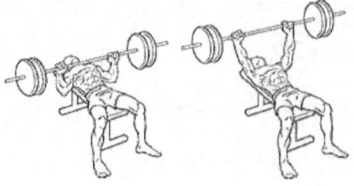

Barbell Bench Chest Press

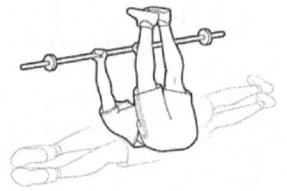

Barbell Floor Wipers

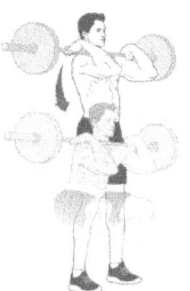

Barbell Front Squat

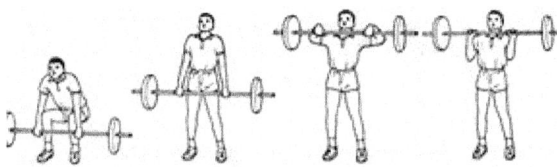

Barbell Power Clean

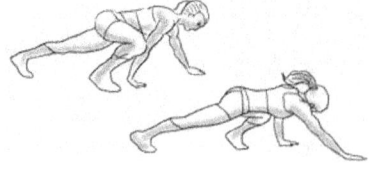

Bear Crawl

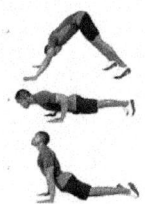

Belly Buster

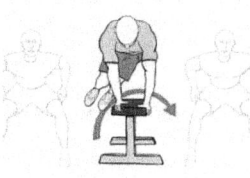

Bench Hop

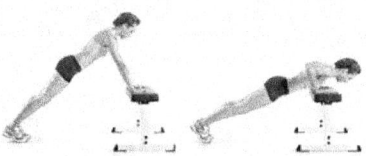

Bench Push-Up

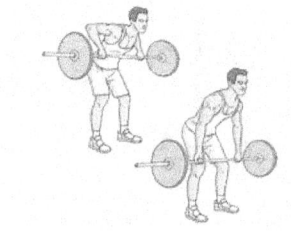

Bend Over Barbell Row

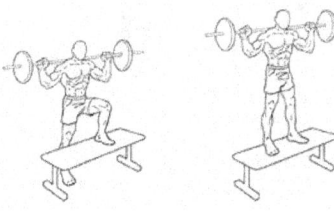

Box or Bench Step-up (Barbell)

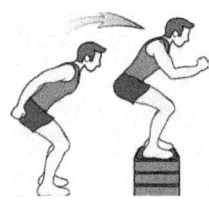

Box Jump

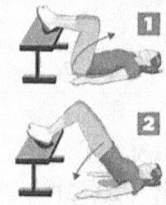

Bridge on Bench

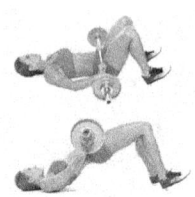

Bridge on Floor with Barbell

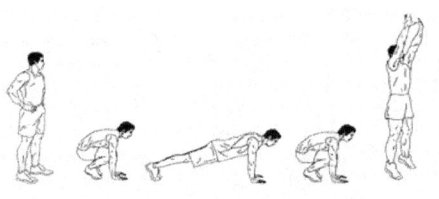

Burpee

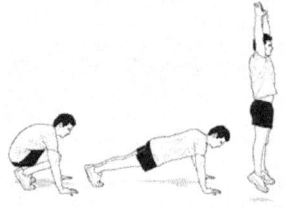 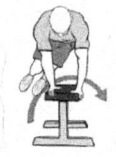

Burpee with Bench Hop

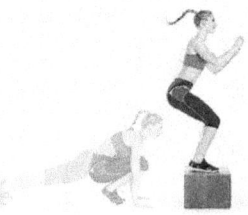

Burpee Jump Box or Bench

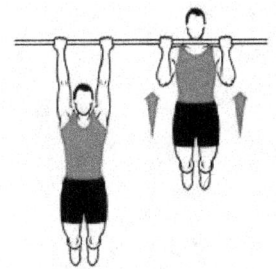

Chin-Up

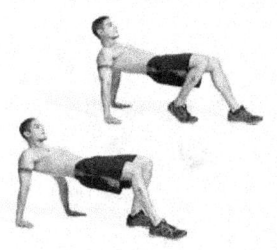

Crab Walk Forward & Backward

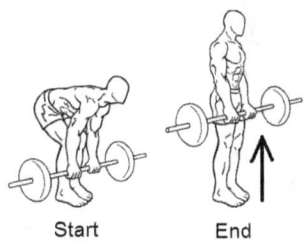

Start   End

Deadlift with Barbell

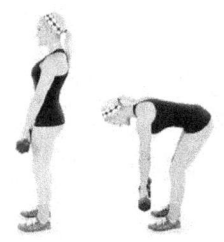

Deadlift with Dumbbells

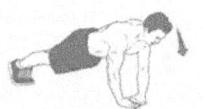

Diamond Push-up

65

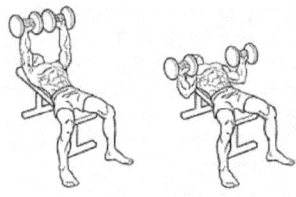

Dumbbells Bench Chest Press

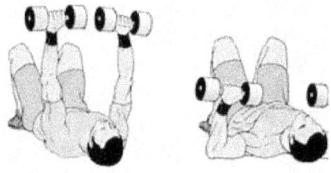

Dumbbells Floor Chest Press

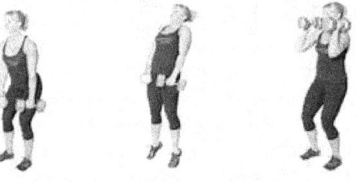

Dumbbells Power Clean

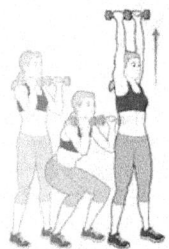

Dumbbells Squat & Press

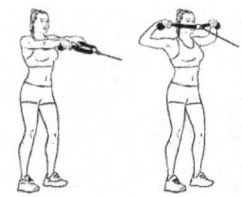

Face Pull (with cable or resistance band)

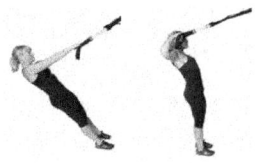

Face Pull (with TRX)

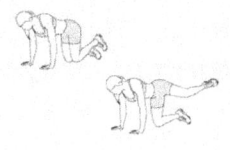

Fire Hydrant

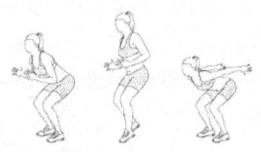

Forward Jump

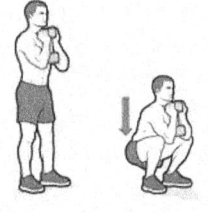

Front Dumbbell Squat

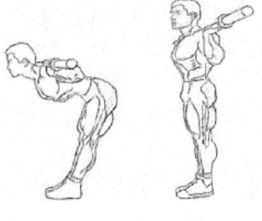

Good Morning (Barbell)

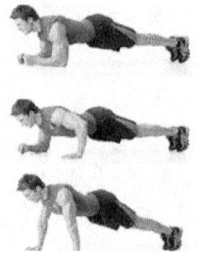

High Low Plank

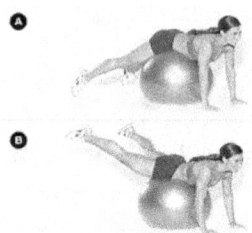

Hip Extension on Stability Ball

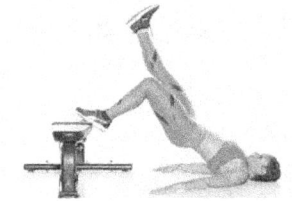

Hip Thrust on Bench – Single Leg

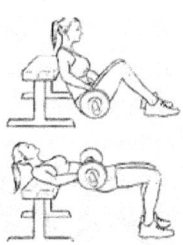

Hip Thrust on Bench (Weight Optional)

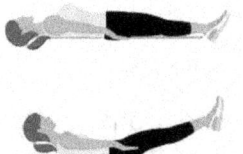

Hollow Hold

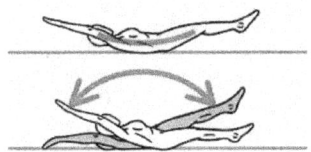

Hollow Rock

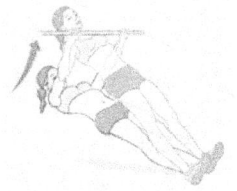

Inverted Row Pull-Up

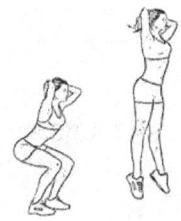

Jump Air Squat

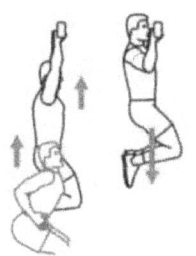

Jumping Pull-up

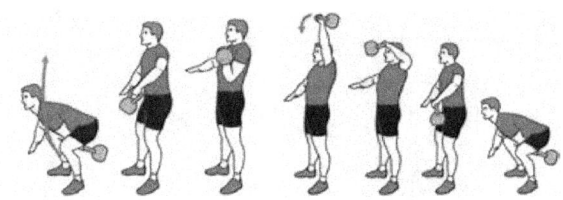

Kettlebell Clean & Press (Single Arm)

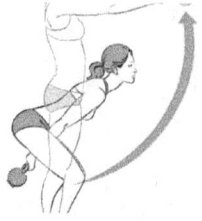

Kettlebell Swing Two Arms

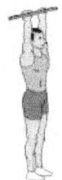 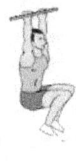 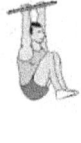

Knees to Elbows

(Modified: Sit on floor, extend legs and arms holding bar, one knee to elbow at a time, alternate)

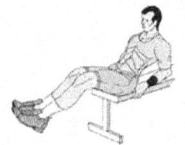 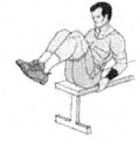

Knee Tuck Crunch on Bench

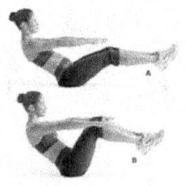

Knee Tuck Crunch on Floor

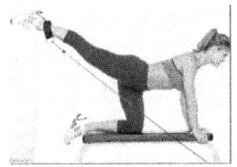

Kneeling Cable Leg Kickback
(Floor or Bench)

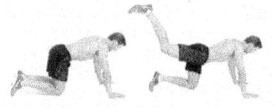

Leg kickback on floor

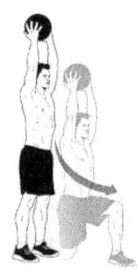

Lunge Overhead Ball

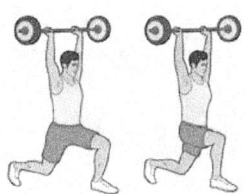

Lunge Overhead Barbell

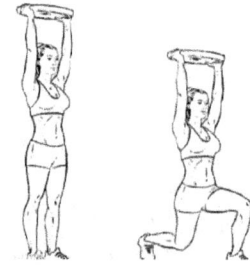

Lunge Plate Weight Overhead

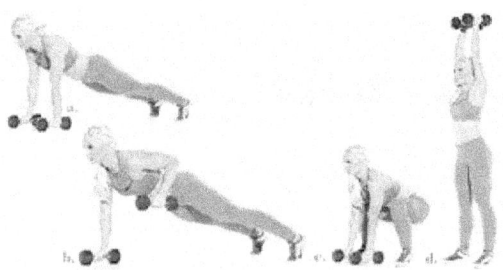

Man Maker

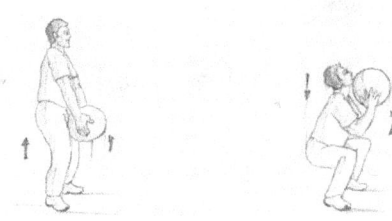

Medicine Ball Clean

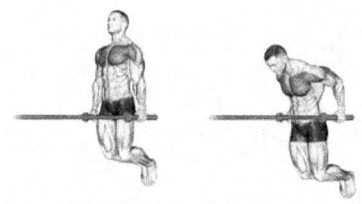

Muscle Up

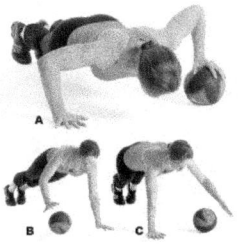

One-Arm Ball Push-Up

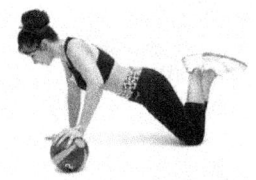

One-Arm Ball Push-Up on Knees

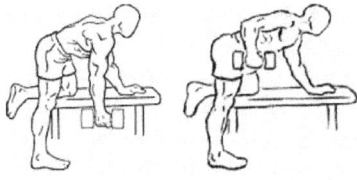

One-Arm Dumbbell Row

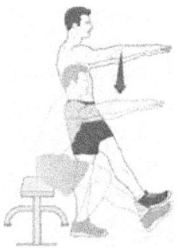

One-Leg Bench Squat

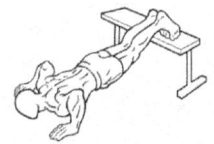

Pike Push-ups on Bench

73

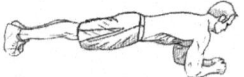

Plank Hold

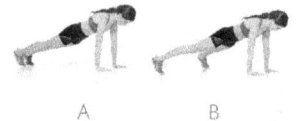

Plank Jack

Plank Knee to Elbow

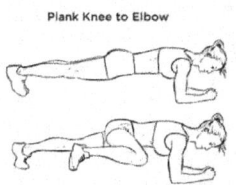

Plank Knee to Elbow

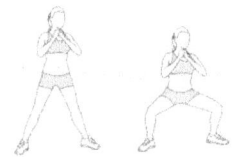

Plie Squat

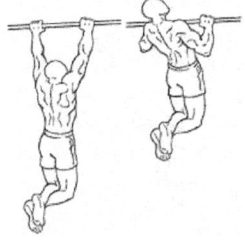

Pull-Up

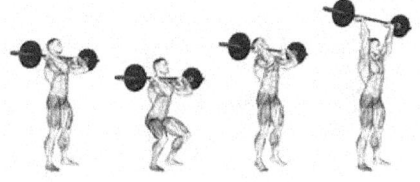

Push Press (Barbell)

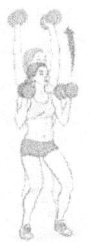

Push Press (Dumbbell)

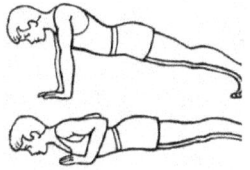

Push-Up

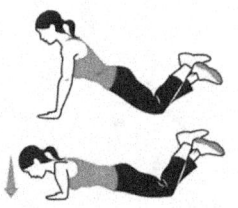

Push-up on Knees

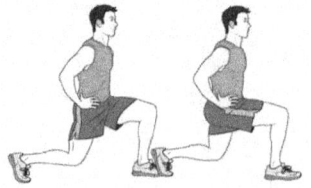

Rear Walking Lunges

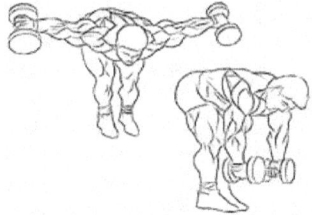

Reverse Fly with Dumbbells

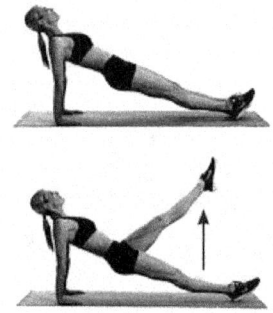

Reverse Plank Kick

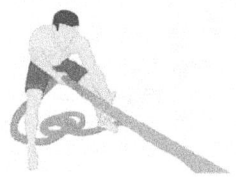

Rope Pull

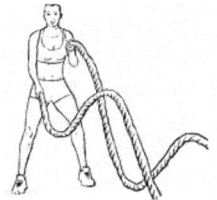

Rope Slam Alternate

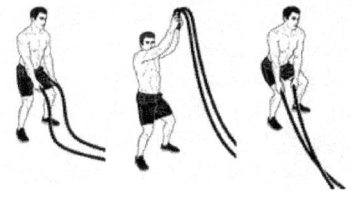

Rope Slam Double Arm

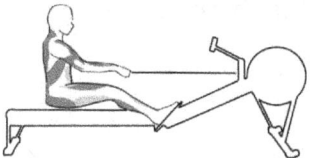

Row

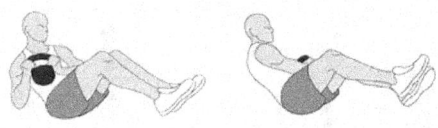

Russian Twist

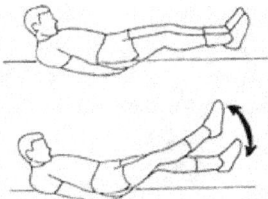

Scissor Kick

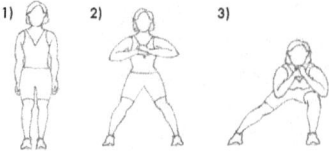

Side Lunge

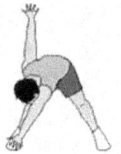

Side Lunge Touch Toes (Alternate)

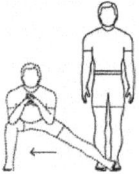

Side Lunge Walking Forward/Backward

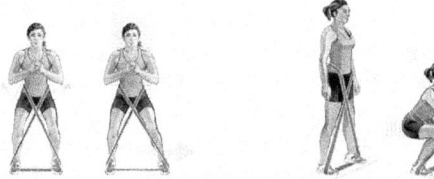

Side Walking Squat with Resistance Band

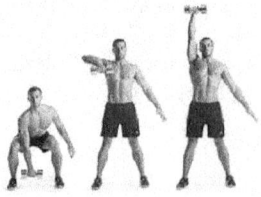

Single-Arm Dumbell Snatch

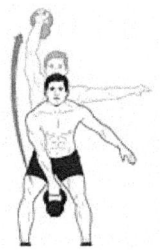

Single-Arm Kettle Bell Swing

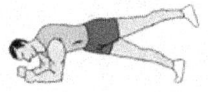

Single Leg Plank

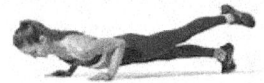

Single Leg Push-Up

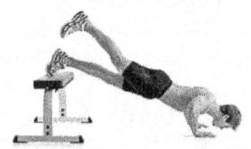

Single Leg Push-up on Bench

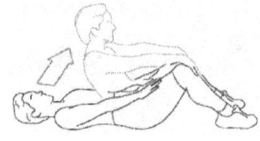

Sit-Up

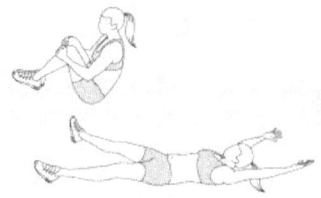

Sit-Up with Knee Tuck with
legs spread apart

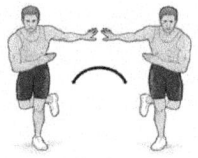

Skater Hop (side to side)

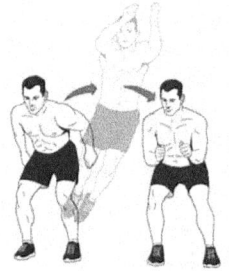

Ski Hop (side to side)

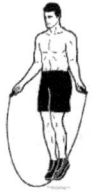

Skip Rope (Modified: skip without rope)

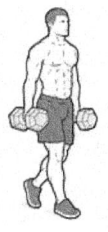

Speed Walk with Dumbbells

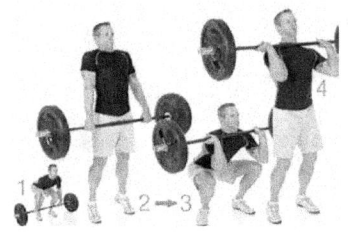

Squat Clean

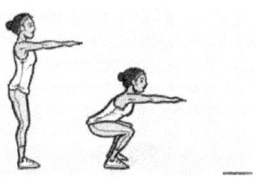

Squat Hold

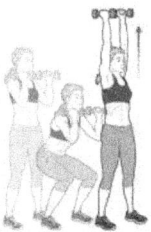

Squat to Overhead Dumbbell Press

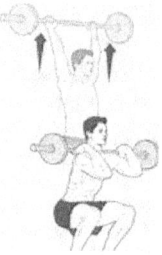

Squat to Overhead Barbell Press

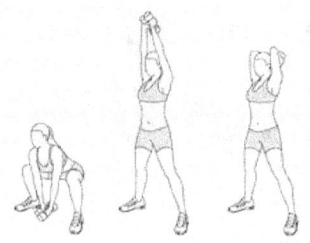

Squat to Overhead Dumbbell Tricep Extension

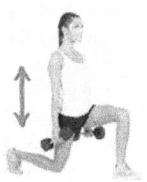

Static Lunge

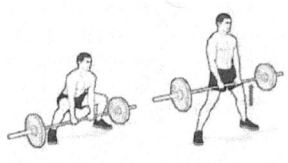

Sumo Deadlift

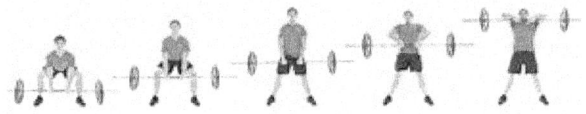

Sumo Deadlift Barbell Upright Row

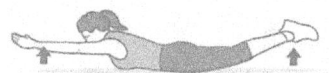

Superman

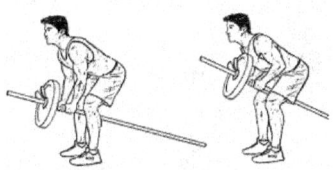

T-Bar Row

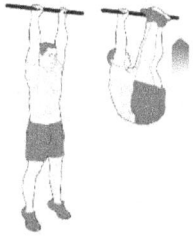

Toes-to-Bar

(Modified: Sit on floor, extend legs and arms holding bar, lift one leg at a time, alternate)

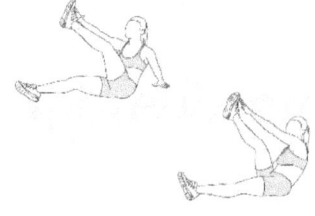

Toes Touch Sit-Up

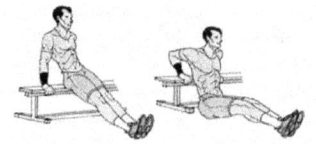

Tricep Dip on Bench

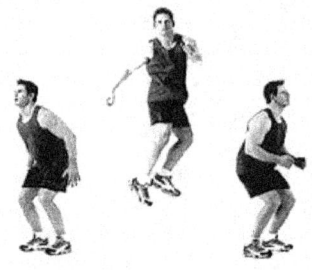

Twisting Jump Squat

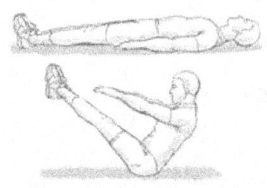

V-Up

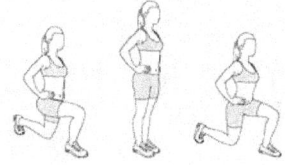

Walking Front Lunge

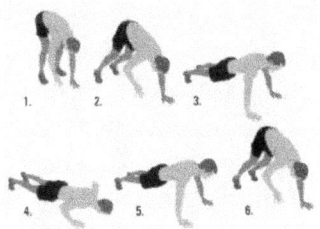

Walking Push-Up

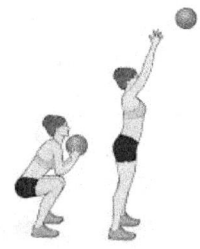

Wall Ball

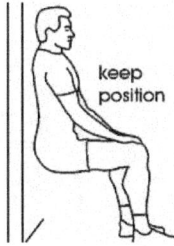

keep
position

Wall Sit (hold position)

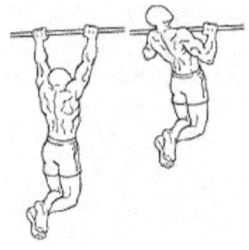

Wide Grip Pull-Up

Designed HIIT Workouts

The following HIIT workouts match the above illustrated exercises which are listed in alphabetical order for an easy search.

There are over 100 workouts to choose from and are designed for beginners to advanced fitness levels.

Performed technique videos can be viewed online.

Here are a few of my suggestions:

1. Make each workout more intense by adding more rounds and/or repetitions.

2. Make them less intense by reducing the number of rounds and/or repetitions.

3. Mix-and-Match exercises and create your own workouts.

Have fun & sweat!

#1
5 Rounds
5 Chin-Ups
15 Air Squats
10 Push-Ups
5 Jump Air Squats
15 **Deadlifts with Dumbbells**
30 Seconds Rest

#2
2 Rounds
16 Box Jumps
16 Jumping Pull-Ups
16 Sit-Ups
16 Kettlebell Swings Two Arms
16 Walking Front Lunges
16 Knees-to-Elbows
16 Push Presses (Barbell)
16 Back Extensions
16 Static Lunges
16 Wall Balls
16 Barbell Floor Wipers
16 Seconds Skip Rope
16 Toes to Bar
1 Minute Rest

#3
3 Rounds
30 Seconds Wall Sit
2 Minutes Run or Speed Walk on Treadmill
12 Single-Arm Kettlebell Swings
12 Ball Squats
12 Twisting Jump Squats
12 Tricep Dips on Bench

12 Supermen
12 Sumo Deadlift
12 Dumbbells Power Cleans
30 Seconds Rest

#4
10-7-5 Reps (Unbreakable)
Squats to Overhead Barbell Presses
Hollow Hold
Dumbbells Floor Chest Presses
Hollow Hold
Diamond Push-ups
Muscle Ups

#5
1 Round
30 Push Presses (Barbell)

#6
4 Rounds
8 Toes-to-Bar or Modified
10 Jump Air Squats
10 Kettle Bell Clean & Press (Single Arm)
20 Rows
8 Arms Dips or Assisted
10 Face Pulls
30 Seconds Rest

#7
4 Rounds
9 Barbell Power Cleans
12 Forward Jumps
9 Deadlifts
12 High Low Planks
9 Static Lunges Each Leg
1 Minute Rest

#8
5 Rounds (Unbreakable)
1 Barbell Power Clean
1 Front Dumbbell Squat
1 Push Press Dumbbells
1 Barbell Back Squat
1 Push Press Dumbbells
1 Sumo Deadlift

#9
6-5-4-3-2-1 Reps
(Unbreakable)
Barbell Bench Chest
    Presses
Deadlifts with Barbell
Inverted Row Pull-Ups
V-Ups
Dumbbells Squat & Press

#10
2 Rounds
1 Minute Wall Balls
1 Minute Skaters
1 Minute Sumo Deadlift
    with Upright Rows
1 Minute Box Jumps
1 Minute Rows
1 Minute Superman Hold
1 Minute Rest

#11
1 Round
20 Air Squats
5 Burpees
30 Sit-Ups
5 Burpees
20 Side Lunges Walking
    Forward/Backward
5 Burpees
15 Kettlebell Cleans &
    Presses
5 Burpees
20 Bear Crawls
5 Burpees
15 Kettlebell Swings
    Two Arms
5 Burpees
20 Side Lunges Walking
    Forward/Backward
5 Burpees
30 Sit-Ups
5 Burpees
15 Deadlifts with
    Dumbbells
20 Air Squats

#12
4 Rounds
20 Rows
10 Dumbbell Squats &
    Presses
10 Walking Push-Ups
30 Seconds Rest

#13
3 Rounds
2 Minute Run Treadmill
  or Speed Walk
12 Each Arm - Kettlebell
  Swings
12 Back Extensions
12 Pull-Ups or Assisted
12 Dumbbells Squat
  & Press
30 Seconds Rest

#14
1 Round
2 Push Press Dumbbells
2 Burpee Bench Jump
  Overs
3 Push Press Dumbbells
3 Burpee Bench Jump
  Overs
4 Push Press Dumbbells
4 Burpee Bench Jump
  Overs
5 Push Press Dumbbells
5 Burpee Bench Jump
  Overs
6 Push Press Dumbbells
6 Burpee Bench Jump
  Overs

#15
3 Rounds
5 Each Single Leg
  Push-Ups
5 **Squats to Overhead
  BB Press**
5 Knees-to-Elbows or
  Modified
5 Deadlifts with Barbell

5 Kettlebell Swings
  Two Arms
5 Chin Ups
5 Good Mornings
5 Face Pulls
5 Forward Jumps
1 Minute Rest

#16
30-20-10 Reps
Ski Jumps
Sit-Ups
Fire Hydrants

#17
3 Rounds
1 Minute Air Bike
20 Medicine Ball Cleans
30 Sit-Ups
20 Bench Push-Ups
30 Air Squats
1 Minute Rest

#18
5 Rounds
3 Squats to Overhead
  DB Press
6 Lunges Barbell
  Overhead
3 Pike Push-Ups on
  Bench
30 Seconds Rest

#19
3 Rounds
2 Man Makers
2 Russian Twists
2 Pull-Ups or Assisted
  Pull-Ups
4 Man Makers
4 Russian Twists
4 Pull-Ups or Assisted
  Pull-Ups
6 Man Makers
6 Russian Twists
6 Pull-Ups or Assisted
  Pull-Ups
1 Minute Rest

#20 (Unbreakable)
20-14-8 Reps
Deadlifts with Barbell
One-Arm Dumbbell Rows
Front Dumbbell Squats
**Dumbbells Floor Chest
  Press**

#21
30 Push Presses
(Barbell)
30 Twisting Jump Squats

#22
50 Wall Balls
30 Toes to Bar
20 **High Low Planks**
15 **Dumbbells Power
  Cleans**

#23
2 Rounds
20 Seconds Skip Rope
  (on toes)
10 Single Arm Dumbbell
  Snatch
20 Seconds Skip Rope
  (on toes)
10 Muscle Ups
20 Seconds Skip Rope
10 Rope Slams Double
  Arms
20 Seconds Skip Rope
10 Dumbbells Squat &
  Press
1 Minute Rest

#24
60 Seconds
Burpees

#25
3 Rounds (Unbreakable)
6 T-Bar Rows
6 Sit-Ups
6 **Diamond Push-ups**
6 Inverted Row Pull-Ups
6 Man Makers
6 **High Low Planks**
6 **Face Pulls**

#26 - 3 Rounds
20 Rope Slams Alternate
20 Lunges Alternate
20 Seconds Single Leg
  Plank (each side)
20 Superman
20 Seconds Wall Sit
1 Minute Rest

#27
2 Rounds
30 Seconds Wall Sit
15 Plank Jacks
30 Lunges Overhead
    Ball (Alternate legs)
15 Jumping Pull-Ups
30 Sit-Ups
15 Good Mornings
1 Minute Rest

#28
2 Rounds
15 Dumbbells Squat
    & Press
15 Bench Hops
20 One-Arm Ball
    Pushups
20 Lunges Overhead
    BB Alternate Legs
30 Scissor Kicks
30 Side Lunges
    Altermate With
    Weights
1 Minute Rest

#29
2 Rounds
10 Jumping Pull-Ups
10 Dumbbells Power
    Cleans
10 Knee Tuck Crunches
    on Floor
10 Walking Push-Ups
30 Seconds Plank Hold
30 Jump Air Squats
1 Minutes Rest

#30
90 Seconds
1 Push Press Dumbbells
1 Burpee
1 Sumo Deadlift BB
    Upright Rows
1 Squat to Overhead
    Tricep Extensions

#31
4 Rounds
5 Squats to Overhead
    Tricep Extensions
5 Hollow Rocks
5 Pull-Ups or Assisted
    Pull-Ups
5 Superman
1 Minute Row
30 Seconds Rest

#32
2-3-4-5-6 Reps
(Unbreakable)
**Squats to Overhead DB
    Presses**
Tricep Dips on Bench
**Dumbbells Floor Chest
    Press**
Burpees Jump Box

#33
30 Reps Each
Barbell Power Cleans
Fire Hydrants
Superman
Squat Hold

#34

1 Round
10 Forward Jumps
10 Jumping Pull-Ups
20 Skater Hops
20 Kettlebell Cleans & Presses
30 Side Lunges Walking Forward/Backward
10 Knees-to-Elbows Pull-ups
30 Skip Rope
15 Push Press Dumbbells
20 Back Extensions
20 Wall Balls
15 Crab Walks
10 Toes Touch Sit-Ups
10 Sumo Deadlifts
10 Static Lunges Each Leg

#35

2 Rounds
15 BoxJumps
15 Kettlebell Cleans & Presses (Single Arm)
20 Barbell Floor Wipers
20 Back Extensions
20 Rope Pulls
20 Toes to Bar
20 Hih Low Planks
Rest 1 minute

#36

2 Rounds
10 Inverted Row Pull-Ups
20 Lunges Plate Weight Overhead (Alternate)
10 Single Leg Push-Ups on Bench (Per Leg)
30 Skip Rope
20 Wall Balls
20 Russian Twists
30 Seconds Wall Sit
Rest 1 minute

#37

3 Rounds
10 Dumbbells Squat & Press
10 Planks Knee to Elbow
20 Walking Front Lunges
30 Seconds Single Leg Plank
30 Seconds Speed Walk with DB
20 Hip Thrusts on Bench Single Leg (Per Leg)
10 Pike Push-Ups on Bench
30 Twisting Jumps Squats
20 Deadlifts with Barbell
10 Static Lunges Each Leg
10 One-Arm Dumbbell Rows
Rest 1 minute

#38
3 Rounds
15 Jump Air Squats
13 Face Pulls
9 Muscle Ups
7 V-Ups
5 Single Arm Dumbbell
   Snatch
Rest 30 Seconds

#39
11-7-5-3 Reps
Ball Squats
Hip Thrusts on Bench
Burpees with Bench
Hops

#40
3 Rounds
12 Toes-to-Bars Alternate
30 Skip Rope
12 Hi Low Planks
12 Squats to Overhead
   Tricep Extensions
Rest 1 minute

#41
2 Rounds
20 Box or Bench
   Step-Ups with Barbell
   Alternate
20 Arm Dips
20 Static Lunges
   (Per Leg)
20 Toes Touch Sit-Ups
1 Minute Rest

#42
5 Rounds
3 Ball Cleans
3 Good Mornings
   (Barbell)
3 Front Dumbbell Squats
30 Seconds Rest

#43
4 Rounds
10 Rope Slams
8 Deadlifts with
   Dumbbells
6 T-Bar Rows
20 Seconds Hollow Holds
10 Forward Jumps
15 Fire Hydrants
30 Seconds Rest

#44
2 Rounds
4 Burpees
4 **Single-Arm Dumbell
   Snatch**
4 Burpees
4 **Single-Arm Dumbell
   Snatch**
4 Burpees
4 **Single-Arm Dumbell
   Snatch**
30 Seconds Plank Hold
1 Minute Rest

#45
1 Round
10 **Pull-ups or Assisted**
20 Push-Ups
20 Air Squats
12 **Pull-ups or Assisted**
15 Push-Ups
25 Jump Air Squats
10 **Pull-ups or Assisted**
15 Push-Ups
20 Air Squats
12 **Pull-ups or Assisted**
20 Pike Push-Ups on
    Bench
25 Plank Jacks
10 Pull-Ups or Assisted
10 Pike Push-Ups on
    Bench
30 Plank Jacks
25 Jump Air Squats

#46
2 Minutes
Dumbbells Carry

#47
3 Rounds
15 **Single-Arm Kettle Bell**
    Swings
20 Seconds Squat Hold
12 Reverse Plank Kicks
    Alternate
20 Lunges Plate Weight
    Overhead (Alternate)
15 Dumbbells Bench
    Chest Press
12 Barbell Front Squats
1 Minute Rest

#48
15-10-7 Reps
(Unbreakable)
Squat Cleans
Face Pulls
Skater Hops
Tricep Dips on Bench

#49
2 Rounds
20 Rows
10 Toes-to-Bars or
    Modified
15 Wall Balls
15 Ball Squat
10 Barbell Power Cleans
20 Skip Rope
10 Muscle Ups
30 Seconds Rest

#50
10-6-2 Reps
(Unbreakable)
Single Arm Dumbell
    Snatch
Burpees
Dumbbells Floor Chest
    Press

#51
5 Rounds
10 Hollow Rocks
10 V-Ups
10 One-Arm Dumbbell
    Rows
10 Seconds Hollow Holds
10 Front Dumbbell
    Squats
1 Minute Rest

#52

15-10-7-3
Back Squat with Barbell
Reverse Flies with
    Dumbbells
Deadlifts with Dumbbells
Inverted Row Pull-Ups
30 Seconds Rest

#53

4 Rounds
30 Skip Rope
15 Push Press
    Dumbbells
10 One-Leg Bench
    Squats Each
15 Fire Hydrants
30 Seconds Rest

#54

3 Rounds
15 Wall Balls
10 Deadlifts with Barbell
10 Dumbbells Power
    Cleans
10 Box Jumps
30 Seconds Rest

#55

15 Unbreakable Reps of
    Each
Kettlebell Swings
    Two-Arms
Box Jumps
Air Squats
Diamond Push-Ups
Knee Tuck Crunches
Burpees
Sit-Ups

Jumping Pull-ups
Skip Rope
Rows
Wall Balls
Back Extensions
Ball Slams
Box or Bench Step-ups
Push Press Dumbbells
Hollow Rocks

#56

5 Rounds
1 Minute Run on Elliptical
10 **Squats to Overhead
    Barbell Press**
1 Minute Rest

#57

5 Rounds
1 Minute Run or Speed
    Walk
10 Ball Slams
10 Box Jumps
10 Wall Balls
10 Jump Air Squats
10 V-Ups
10 Dumbbells Squat &
    Press
30 Seconds Rest

#58
2 Rounds (unbreakable)
10 Deadlifts with Barbell
10 Box Jumps
10 Kettlebell Cleans &
   Presses
10 Knees-to-Elbows
10 Sit-Ups
10 Jumping Pull-Ups
10 Hip Thrusts on
   Bench (Per Leg)
10 Dumbbells Squat &
   Press
10 Skip Rope
10 Ball Slams (as far as
   you can)
10 Superman
10 Dumbbells Power
   Cleans
10 Burpees
1 Minute Rest

#59 -
4 Rounds
16 Rope Slams Alternate
30 Skip Rope
16 Dumbbells Bench
   Chest Press
30 Seconds Rest

#60 - 4 Rounds
5 Single Leg Push-Ups
   (Per Leg)
10 One-Leg Bench
   Squats (Alternate
   Legs)
10 Sumo Deadlifts
10 Chin-Ups
30 Seconds Rest

#61
1 Round
10 Box Jumps
20 Seconds Speed Walk
   with Heavy Dumbbells
10 Single-Arm Kettle Bell
   Swings
20 Seconds Speed Walk
   with Heavy Dumbbells
10 Squat to Overhead BB
   Press
10 Box Jumps
20 Seconds Speed Walk
   with Heavy Dumbbells
10 Inverted Row Pullups
20 Seconds Speed Walk
   with Heavy Dumbbells
10 Box Jumps
20 Seconds Speed Walk
   with Heavy Dumbbells
10 Squat to Overhead
   Dumbbell Tricep
   Extension
20 Seconds Speed Walk
   with Heavy Dumbbells

#62
2 Rounds
20 Muscle Ups
60 Seconds Wall Sit
20 High Low Planks
20 Forward Jumps
20 Face Pulls

#63
1 Round
4 Burpees Bench Jump
  Over
20 Rows
4 Burpees Bench Jump
  Over
10 Wall Balls
4 Burpees Bench Jump
  Over
20 Deadlifts with Barbell
4 Burpees Bench Jump
  Over
10 Single Leg Push-Ups
  (Per Leg)
4 Burpees Bench Jump
  Over
20 Bear Crawls
4 Burpees Bench Jump
  Over

#64
4 Rounds (Unbreakable)
6 Jump Air Squats
12 Rear Walking Lunges
6 **Dumbbells Floor Chest
Press**
6 Burpees
12 Toes to Bar
6 Dumbbells Squat &
Press

#65
2 Rounds
15 Wall Balls
30 Skip Rope
15 Box Jumps
10 Toes-to-Bars
10 Inverted Row Pullups

10 Twisting Jump Squats
10 Barbell Power Cleans
10 Hip Thrusts on Bench
  Single Leg
10 Medicine Ball Cleans
10 Side Lunges Walking
  Forward/Backward
1 Minute Rest

#66
4 Rounds (Unbreakable)
7 Back Extensions
7 Pull-Ups or Assisted
Pull-Ups
7 Ski Hops
7 **Dumbbells Bench
  Chest Press**

#67
2 Rounds
20 T-Bar Rows
20 One-Leg Bench
  Squats (Alternate)
20 Sumo Deadlift Barbell
  Upright Rows
20 Hollow Holds
20 Squats to Overhead
  Dumbbell Presses
20 Sit-Ups with Knee
  Tucks
20 Push Press
  Dumbbells
1 Minute Rest

#68
1 Round
4 Burpees
3 Push-Ups
3 Barbell Power Cleans
6 One-Arm Ball
  Push-Ups Alternate
3 Barbell Power Cleans
6 Push-Ups
3 Barbell Power Cleans
9 Bench Push-Ups
6 Barbell Power Cleans
9 Pike Push-Ups on
  Bench
6 Barbell Power Cleans
6 Walking Push-Ups
9 Barbell Power Cleans
3 Diamond Push-Ups
9 Barbell Power Cleans

#69
4 Rounds
10 Single Arm Dumbbell
  Snatch
8 Side Lunges Touch
  Toes (Alternate)
6 Muscle Ups
10 Fire Hydrants
30 Seconds Rest

#70
2 Rounds
2 Minute Rows
12 Sumo Deadlifts
  Barbell Upright Rows
20 Box Jumps
1 Minute Rest

#71
8-6-4-2 Reps
Muscle Ups
Dumbbells Power Cleans
Toes Touch Sit-Ups
Squat Cleans (Barbell)
30 Seconds Rest

#72
3 Rounds
1 Minute Air Bike
6 High Low Planks
12 Good Mornings
  (Barbell)
6 Reverse Flies
  (Dumbbell)
12 Twisting Jump Squats
12 Tricep Dips on Bench
12 Toes Touch Sit-Ups
30 Seconds Rest

#73
3 Rounds
15 Sumo Deadlifts
  Barbell Upright Rows
20 Side Lunges
  (Alternate)
20 Rope Pulls
20 Sit-ups
10 One-Arm Ball
  Push-Ups
10 Air Squats
1 Minute Rest

#74
4 Rounds
10 Superman
10 Ball Slams
5 Barbell Front Squats
5 Push Presses (Barbell)
5 Barbell Back Squats
10 V-Ups
10 One-Arm Dumbbell
  Rows
5 **Dumbbells Bench
  Chest Press**
1 Minute Rest

#75
2 Rounds
20 Single-Arm Kettlebell
  Swings
20 Forward Single-Leg
  Jumps (10 each leg)
20 Knee Tuck Crunches
  on Bench
20 Lunges Overhead
  Barbell (Alternate)
10 Crab Walk Forward
10 Crab Walk Backward
20 Jump Air Squats
1 Minute Rest

#76
2 Rounds
30 Rows
30 Skater Hops
15 **Dumbbells Floor
Chest Press**
30 Supermen
30 Face Pulls
2 Minutes Air Bike
1 Minute Rest

#77
3 Rounds
1 Deadlift with Barbell
  (as heavy as you can)
2 Forward Jumps
3 One-Leg Bench Squats
  (Per Leg)
4 High Low Planks
5 Squat Cleans
6 Sit-Ups
7 Muscle Ups
8 Dumbbells Squat &
  Press
30 Seconds Rest

#78
1 Round
4 Deadlifts with Barbell
4 Box Jumps
6 Deadlifts with Barbell
6 Box Jumps
8 Deadlifts with Barbell
8 Box Jumps
10 Deadlifts with Barbell
10 Box Jumps
12 Deadlifts with Barbell
12 Box Jumps
14 Deadlifts with Barbell
14 Box Jumps

#79
2 Rounds
12 Pull-Ups or Assisted
   Pull-ups
16 Back Extensions
20 Pike Push-Ups on
   Bench
12 Box Jumps
16 **Dumbbells Bench**
   Chest Press
20 Barbell Floor Wipers
12 Man Makers
1 Minute Rest

#80
1 Round
1 Minute Weighted
  Walk/Run
20 Deadlifts with Barbell
1 Minute Weighted
  Walk/Run
20 One-Arm Ball
   Push-Ups Alternate
1 Minute Weighted
  Walk/Run
20 Ball Squats
1 Minute Weighted
  Walk/Run
20 Push Presses
   (Barbell)
1 Minute Weighted
  Walk/Run

#81
5-10-1-20-25-20-15-10-5
Reps
Skip Rope

#82
1 Round
1 Minute Run
12 Single Arm Dumbbell
   Snatch
12 Box Jumps
12 Pull-Ups or Assisted
   Pull-Ups
12 Barbell Back Squats
12 Medicine Ball Cleans
12 Air Squats
12 High Low Planks
12 Side Lunges
12 Wall Balls
12 Deadlifts with Barbell
12 Lunges Overhead
   Plate Weight
   (Alternate)
12 Rope Slam Alternate
12 Bear Crawls
12 Sumo Deadlift Barbell
   Upright Rows
12 Box or Bench
   Step-Ups (Barbell)
12 Bend Over Barbell
   Rows
12 Push-Ups
12 Inverted Row Pull-Ups
12 Skater Hops
12 Ball Slams
12 Burpee Jump Box or
   Bench
12 V-Ups
12 Rope Pulls
12 Walking Front Lunges
12 Kettlebell Cleans &
   Presses
12 Tricep Dips on Bench

#83
1 Round
12 Burpees
1 Minute Run
20 Push-Ups
1 Minute Run
30 Walking Lunges
1 Minute Run
12 Medicine Ball Cleans
30 Air Squats
1 Minute Run
12 Jumping Pull-Ups
30 Walking Lunges
1 Minute Run
20 One-Arm Ball
   Push-Ups
   (Alternate)
1 Minute Run
12 V-Ups
12 Toes to Bar

#84
3 Rounds (Unbreakable)
8 Dumbbells Power
   Cleans
7 Sumo Deadlifts
6 Walking Push-Ups
5 Man Makers
4 Air Squats
3 Diamond Push-Ups
2 Bridges on Bench
1 Chin Up

#85
1 Round
24 Air Squats
24 Push-Ups
24 Side Lunges Walking
   Forward/Backward
24 Crab Walks
   Forward/Backward
2 Minute Run or Speed
   Walk

#86
3 Rounds
30 Seconds Wall Sit
30 Seconds Plank Hold
8 Back Extension
8 Front Dumbbell Squats
8 Inverted Row Pull-Ups
8 Skater Hops
8 Deadlifts with Barbell
8 Rope Pulls
8 Static Lunges Each Leg
8 Sit-Ups
8 Box Jumps
8 V-Ups
8 Walking Push-Up
8 Bend Over Barbell
   Rows
8 Fire Hydrants
1 Minute Rest

#87
2 Rounds
3 Barbell Power Cleans
3 Barbell Front Squats
6 Barbell Power Cleans
6 Toes-to-Bars
9 Box Jumps
9 Toes to Bars
12 Box Jumps
12 Toes to Bars
1 Minute Rest

#88
3 Rounds
9 Burpees
9 Good Mornings
9 Box Jumps
9 Medicine Ball Cleans
9 Toes to Bar
9 Lunges Overhead
  Barbell
9 Knee Tuck Crunches
  on Floor
30 Seconds Rest

#89
3 Rounds
10 Medicine Ball Cleans
30 Skip Rope
15 Wall Balls
12 Hip Thrusts on Bench
10 Sumo Deadlifts
30 Seconds Rest

#90
30 seconds rest between
  sets
40 T-Bar Rows
30 Twisting Jump Squats
20 Wall Balls
20 Russian Twists with
  Ball
20 Ball Slams
20 Sit-Ups with Ball

#91
2 Rounds
8 Man Makers
20 Seconds Plank Hold
20 Deadlifts with Barbell
20 Seconds Wall Sit
20 One-Arm Dumbbell
  Rows
20 Jump Air Squats
20 Scissor Kicks
20 Static Lunges
  (each leg)
1 Minute Rest

#92
1 Round
50 Skip Rope
50 Rows
30 Face Pulls
20 Dumbbells Squat &
  Press

#93
4 Rounds
6 Inverted Row Pull-Ups
6 Squat Cleans
6 **Dumbbells Bench
Chest Press**
12 Scissor Kicks
30 Seconds Rest

#94
3 Rounds
14 Russian Twists
12 Deadlifts with
   Dumbbells
10 Hollow Rocks
9 Barbell Power Cleans
8 Lunges Plate Weight
   Overhead (Alternate)
6 Push Presses (Barbell)
30 Seconds Rest

#95
3 Rounds
15 Box Jumps
12 Dumbbells Floor
   Chest Press
9 Toes to Bars
6 Barbell Arm Curls
5 Supermen
30 Seconds Rest

#96 - 10-8-4 Reps
      (Unbreakable)
Pike Push-Ups on Bench
Hip Thrusts on Bench
Arm Dips or Assisted
Rear Walking Lunges
Muscle Ups
Air Squats

#97
5 Rounds (Unbreakable)
2 Medicine Ball Cleans
3 (Each Leg) Box/Bench
   Step-Ups
4 Diamond Push-Ups
5 One-Leg each Bench
   Squats
6 Inverted Row Pull-Ups
15 Skip Rope

#98 - 2 Rounds
20 Box/Bench Step-Ups
   with Barbell
   (Alternate Leg)
12 Barbell Power Cleans
20 Box/Bench Step-Ups
   with Barbell Alternate
12 Single Arm Dumbbell
   Snatch
1 Minute Rest

#99 - 2 Rounds
90 Seconds Rear
   Walking Lunges with
   Dumbbells
15 Assisted Pull-Ups
16 Seconds Hollow Holds
8 Dumbbells Power
   Cleans

#100
3 Rounds
2 minutes Air Bike
1 minute Rest
2 minutes Rows
1 minute Rest
2 minutes Ski Hops
1 minute Rest

#101
2 Rounds
10 Kettle Bell Clean &
    Press (light weight)
    (single arm)
10 Kettle Bell Clean &
    Press (medium
    weight) (single arm)
10 Kettle Bell Clean &
    Press (heavy weight)
    (single arm)
10 Kettle Bell Clean &
    Press (max weight)
    (single arm)
1 Minute Rest

#102
4 Rounds
15 T-Bar Rows
15 Superman
30 Seconds Rest

#103
3 Rounds
15 Wall Balls
10 Sumo Deadlift Upright
    Rows
10 Box Jumps
10 Face Pulls
30 Rows
20 Bench Push-Ups
10 Barbell Back Squats
1 Minute Rest

CORE

#104
4 Rounds
30 Seconds Plank Hold
15 Scissor Kicks
15 Plank Jacks
10 Russian Twists
10 Planks Knee to Elbow
30 Seconds Rest

#105
3 Rounds
12 Sit-Ups
12 Reverse Plank Kicks
12 Sit-Ups with Knee
    Tucks
12 Single Leg Planks
12 Toes Touch Sit-Ups
1 Minute Speed Walk
    with DB
30 Seconds Rest

#106 - 4 Rounds
6 Superman
6 V-Ups
6 Wall Sit
6 Back Extensions
6 Ball Slams
No Rest

#107 - 4 Rounds
8 Toes to Bar Alternate
8 Belly Busters
8 Barbell Floor Wipers
16 Bear Crawls
8 Bridges on Bench
8 Knees to Elbows
No Rest

#108
3 Rounds
20 Crab Walks
10 Hip Thrusts on Bench
    Single Leg
20 Rope Pulls
10 Single Leg Push-Ups
    (Per Leg)
20 Squat Hold
10 Man Makers
30 Seconds Rest

#109
4 Rounds
15 Seconds Hollow Holds
10 High/Low Planks
10 Hollow Rocks
10 Knee Tuck Crunches
30 Seconds Rest

#110
4 Rounds
10 Bridges on Bench
10 Belly Buster
10 Sit-Ups with Knee
    Tucks
10 Scissor Kicks
30 Seconds Rest

#111
5 Rounds
5 Back Extensions
5 Sit-Ups
5 Planks Knee to Elbows
5 Wall Sits
5 Ball Slams
5 Man Makers
5 Push-Ups
No Rest

#112
4 Rounds
10 V-Ups
20 Bear Crawls
10 Reverse Plank Kicks
10 Superman
30 Seconds Rest

#113
3 Rounds
20 Rope Pulls
20 Plank Jacks
20 Hip Thrusts on Bench
20 Toes to Bar Alternate
1 Minute Rest

#114
4 Rounds
10 Hollow Rocks
10 Reverse Plank Kicks
10 Russian Twists
10 Barbell Floor Wipers
30 Seconds Rest

#115 – 1 Round (Unbreakable)
4 Rope Slams Double
   Arms
4 Scissor Kicks
4 Plank Jacks
4 Russian Twists
4 Man Makers
4 Knees to Elbows
4 Reverse Plank Kicks
4 Single Leg Planks
4 Sit-Ups with Knee
   Tucks
4 Toes Touch Sit-Ups
4 Superman
4 V-Ups
4 Toes to Bar Alternate
4 Back Extensions
4 Ball Slams
4 Belly Buster
4 Bear Crawls
4 Barbell Floor Wipers
4 Bridges on Bench
4 Crab Walks
4 Hip Thrusts on Bench
4 Hollow Rocks
4 High/Low Planks
4 Knee Tuck Crunches
4 Rope Slams Alternate

#116 - 1 Round (Unbreakable)
40 Sit-Ups
40 Knee Tuck Crunches

#117
2 Rounds
30 V-Ups
30 Supermen
30 Squat Hold
1 Minute Rest

#118
2 Rounds
30 Russian Twists
30 Belly Busters
30 Seconds Rest

#119
1 Round (Unbreakable)
40 Hip Thrusts on Bench
40 Wall Sits
20 Single Leg Planks
   (Per Leg)

#120
2 Rounds
40 Plank Jacks
20 Ball Slams
1 Minute Rest

#121
3 Rounds
5 Single Leg Push-Ups
   on Bench (Per Leg)
10 Sit-Ups with Knee
   Tucks
20 Planks Knee to Elbow
   Alternate
5 Man Makers
10 Knees to Elbows

GLUTES & HIP FLEXORS

#121
2 Rounds
20 Side Walking Squats
   With Resistance
   Bands (each side)
20 Leg Kickbacks on
   Floor (Per Leg)
20 Fire Hydrants
   (Per Leg)
20 Plie Squats

#122
3 Rounds
20 Kneeling Cable Leg
   Kickbacks (Per Leg)
20 Bridges on Floor
20 **Hip Extensions on
   Stability Ball**
30 Seconds Rest

#123
4 Rounds
20 Plie Squats
20 Fire Hydrants
   (Per Leg)
20 Bridges on Floor with
   Barbell
30 Seconds Rest

#124
4 Rounds
20 Leg Kickbacks on
   Floor (Per Leg)
10 Side Walking Squats
   With Resistance
   Bands (each side)
15 **Hip Extensions on
   Stability Ball**
30 Seconds Rest

#125
4 Rounds
20 Fire Hydrants
   (Per Leg)
20 Bridges on Floor with
   Barbell
30 Seconds Rest

#126
4 Rounds
10 Side Walking Squats
   With Resistance
   Bands (each side)
20 Plie Squats
10 Kneeling Cable Leg
   Kickbacks (Per Leg)
No Rest

CARDIO & WARM-UP

#127
30 Skater Hops (side to
    side)
30 Ski Hops (side to side)
30 Skip Rope
    (Modified: without
        rope)

#128
30 Jumping Jacks
30 Plank Jacks
30 Jump Air Squats

#129
1 Minute Running in
    place
10 Burpees
3 Minute Run on
    Treadmill High Speed
5 Burpees

#130
1 Minute Eliptical
10 Rounds Short Sprints
1 Minute Eliptical
8 Rounds Short Sprints
1 Minute Eliptical
6 Rounds Short Sprints
1 Minutes Eliptical
4 Rounds Short Sprints

In Summary

Physical exercise is widely recognized as the best way to keep the body healthy and active. Neglect of bodily health can be disastrous for us. It causes several physical and mental problems. Slowly our body becomes vulnerable to many diseases. His energy and beauty is lost early. He grows old early. Strength, stamina and power of concentration decline.

Physical exercise is of different kind. Different people have different choices and preferences. Many people enjoy morning walk. Some find pleasure in cycling and jogging. Several people like to do gardening or swimming. Many people find it easier and convenient to spend an hour or two in doing workout in a well-equipped gym. Skipping is also a popular way to keep one's body fit and healthy. These days' yoga and meditation are also gaining popularity. They are easier to practice and highly effective in keeping one fit and healthy.

Regularity in exercise is imperative for the preservation of good health. It is a good source of energy, stamina and strength. Consistency adds to the result of exercise. Lack of it cannot bring good result. So, we should be very regular and consistent in physical exercise.

Physical exercise is a form of discipline. It means self-control and sincerity. We need to neglect our idleness. Physical exercise helps in character building. It makes our mind sharp and active. It improves mental strength and capability. It adds to our capability and improves our performance. Physical exercise done in morning keeps us healthy, fit and active for the whole day, therefore, we should do it regularly. It is a must to keep us fit and healthy.

No Excuses!

My Book References

. **You will see it when you believe it**
   2018 on Amazon.com

. **You're Worth It**
   2019 on Amazon.com

Health & Fitness Coach
Certified Personal Trainer, CFPA
Fitness Instructor and Nutrition Specialist, ICSC
Certified Kickboxing Instructor, FKC
Certified Reiki Master & Teacher
Certified Intuitive Energy Channeler
Certified Hypnosis Therapy
Certified Crystal Healing Therapy
Certified Chi Gong Instructor
Freelance Writer

*For any requests on nutrition plan, personal training programs
and coaching, please contact me at (416) 388-2541 or
lapierresuzie6@gmail.com*

facebook.com/risebright&fit
suziehealing.com